COLUMBIA COLLEGE LIBRARY
600 S. MICHIGAN AVENUE
CHICAGO, IL 60605

COLUMBIA COLLEGE CHICAGO
3 2711 00164 5849

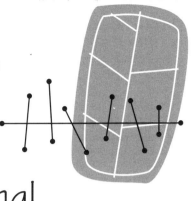

Active Interventions for Kids and Teens: Adding Adventure and Fun to Counseling!

Jeffrey S. Ashby, PhD
Terry Kottman, PhD
Donald DeGraaf, PhD

D1609635

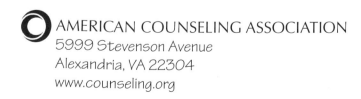

AMERICAN COUNSELING ASSOCIATION
5999 Stevenson Avenue
Alexandria, VA 22304
www.counseling.org

ENTERED MAR 1 0 2010

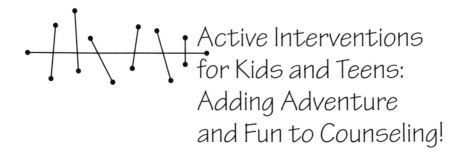

Active Interventions
for Kids and Teens:
Adding Adventure
and Fun to Counseling!

Copyright © 2008 by the American Counseling Association. All rights reserved. Printed in the United States of America. Except as permitted under the United States Copyright Act of 1976, no part of this publication may be reproduced or distributed in any form or by any means, or stored in a database or retrieval system, without the written permission of the publisher.

10   9   8   7   6   5   4   3   2   1

American Counseling Association
5999 Stevenson Avenue
Alexandria, VA 22304

Director of Publications • Carolyn C. Baker

Production Manager • Bonny E. Gaston

Copy Editor • Lucy Blanton

Editorial Assistant • Catherine A. Brumley

Cover and text design by Bonny E. Gaston.

Library of Congress Cataloging-in-Publication Data

Ashby, Jeffrey S.
    Active interventions for kids and teens: adding adventure and fun to counseling!/Jeffrey S. Ashby, Terry Kottman and Donald DeGraaf.
        p. ; cm.
    Includes bibliographical references.
    ISBN 978-1-55620-256-8 (alk. paper)
    1. Adventure therapy for children.   I. Kottman, Terry.   II. DeGraaf, Donald G.   III. Title.
    [DNLM: 1. Child.   2. Play Therapy—methods.   3. Adolescent.   4. Behavior Therapy.   WS 350.2
A823a 2008]
    RJ505.A38A84 2008
    618.92'891653—dc22   2007045521

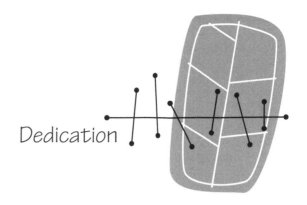

Dedication

It's pretty much always, and for too many reasons to list, to Lucy, Samuel, John, Elizabeth, and Isaac; Kathy, Isaac, and Rochelle; Jacob and Rick. It's also to all the Adventurers in classes and workshops over the years at Georgia State University, the University of Northern Iowa, Calvin College, and the Hong Kong Adventure Therapy Institute. Thanks to all of you for sharing adventures with us!

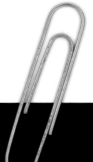

Table of Contents

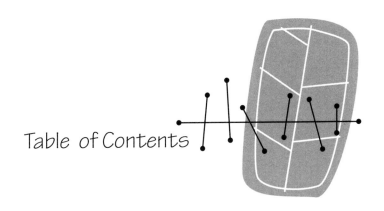

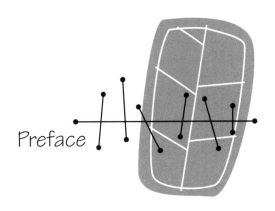

Preface

Hey, thanks for reading the preface. Not everybody does, and we appreciate it. We've written this book for several reasons. One reason is that we had a lot of fun writing a similar book designed specifically for school counselors working with Grades K–8 (*Adventures in Guidance*). We've had a great response to that book and have been asked, "Do you have any other activities?" "Do you have any activities for older kids or adults?" or "Do you have another activity for _____?" Our answer is nearly always "yes," or in rare cases, "Not off the top of my head, but I know that Jeff, Terry, or Don does. I'll ask!" This book contains some of those other activities. These are not our second tier activities (ones that didn't make the cut in the other book we did together). This book contains some of our favorites, and many of the ones we use most often. This book also includes activities that fit well for youth older than Grade 8 and adults. A second reason we've written this book is because we want to promote the value for counselors, therapists, and psychologists of having more FUN! We think that these activities can be FUN and that that fun can actually facilitate the learning, development, insight, and change we're trying to facilitate in our clients. A third reason we wrote this book is because we think that the use of these activities really can accomplish the goals and objectives you have for your clients. These goals and objectives are consistent with typical mental health objectives and reflect traditional guidance curriculum goals used by school counselors.

The book is organized such that it can be read straight through, though we think it is highly unlikely that most people will do this. (Please do consider this a challenge/invitation to be one of those select few.) The bulk of the book (chapter 7) describes 50 activities that can be led and facilitated to accomplish specific goals and objectives. We anticipate that many folks will move to Appendix B, which organizes the 50 activities by goals, objectives, and grade levels. In this way, if you are really interested in helping your clients "express feelings clearly and constructively" and "recognize and accept the feelings of others," you can move to the section of the grid identifying those goals and objectives and be led to numerous activities that can be facilitated to meet these goals. Each activity description explains what to do in the activity, what the ideal size group might be (e.g., 2, maybe just you and the client, to 100!), any materials needed and preparation, and any safety concerns ("You'll shoot your eye out!"). Further, each activity has a list of processing questions that can help you bridge from the activity to a productive processing discussion. In short, we wrote this book for you to USE. If you never read the chapters, we'll get over it. But if the book sits on your shelf, we'll be deeply disappointed, maybe even wounded. (But don't take this guilt on!)

In addition to the activities and the appendixes organizing activities by goals, objectives, and activity types, we've written six scintillating chapters. We think of these chapters as "What You Need to Know Before You Play." In chapter 1, we briefly discuss the rationale for using games and adventure therapy intervention strategies as a therapeutic modality with children and teens. We also discuss the four categories or forms of games and activities included in the book and when and how you might want to use them.

In chapter 2 we discuss the practical factors relevant to using adventure activities with children and teens. If you'd like to review some developmental considerations in treatment planning with children and adolescents, this is a chapter to read!

Chapter 3 discusses the practicalities of leading these activities in ways that are safe, facilitative of the goals, and fun. We address all sorts of questions, such as, "Do you play also or just lead and watch?"

In chapter 4 we dig into processing adventure activities. We discuss a variety of ideas for processing insights developed during the game playing and for helping participants generalize these insights into other relationships and situations.

Chapter 5 provides guidelines for using and adapting the various activities described in this book, and chapter 6 explains in greater depth how to use the activities. We discuss each component of the template used to organize the lessons, how the activities are grouped relative to guidance and treatment goals and objectives, and how they can be cross-referenced and used to meet several different objectives at the same time across components.

You obviously will move to the sections and chapters of the book that meet your needs. We've tried to be practical, and we've tried to have fun. We trust that you will do the same—and have FUN USING the book!

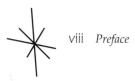

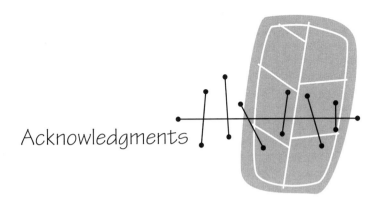

Acknowledgments

Coming up with documentation for all of the sources for the ideas and activities in this book was almost impossible. We all know a LOT of activities, and trying to figure out the who and where of when we first learned every single activity was daunting. So, if we know where we got an activity, we have tried to give credit to that specific source. Many times, though, all three of us knew an activity and learned it in very different places. That is the nature of adventure education and adventure therapy. However, we do know some of the people who came before us and helped us to get to the place where we could write this book and teach these activities, and we want to acknowledge them: Craig Anderson, Jim Cain, Wendy Dickinson, Jeff Goldberg, Arlene Hess, John Krafka, Deb Jordan, Jim Martin, Ann McElfresh, Mike McGowen, Karl Rohnke, Stuart Shepley, Jennifer Stewart, Kris Terry, Sue Walden, and Bradford Woods; and Camp Adventure, Project Adventure, the New Games Foundation, and the North Carolina Outward Bound School.

We want to thank a slew of folks who helped along the way—figuring out how to make our computers talk to one another, reading activities to make sure that they made sense, testing out activities and processing questions to see that they would work with kids: Lucy Ashby, Rick Kottman, Andrea Christopher, and all of the fifth graders in Cedar Falls, Iowa, and the sixth graders at Lincoln Elementary and North Cedar Elementary. We would also like to thank our editor, Carolyn Baker, for her expertise and generosity of spirit, but most of all for her patience. Any activities that do not make sense or do not work the way we have described them or processing questions that fall flat are purely the problem of the authors, not these dedicated, helpful, and fun individuals.

Thanks to Emily, Tim, Leah, Dawn, and all the other baristas at Cup of Joe in Cedar Falls, Iowa for providing me with what I needed to get through writing my part of the book.

—TK

.

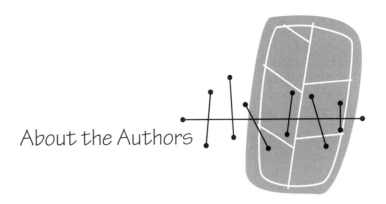

About the Authors

Jeffrey S. Ashby, PhD, ABPP, is a professor of counseling psychology at Georgia State University in Atlanta, Georgia. He is the former director of the counseling psychology PhD program at Georgia State. Jeff has written and presented in the areas of counseling, perfectionism, and stress. He has a consulting practice and lives in Atlanta with his wife Lucy and his four children, Isaac, Eliza, John, and Samuel (a constant adventure!).

Terry Kottman, PhD, NCC, RPT-S, LMHC, founded The Encouragement Zone, a center where she provides play therapy training, counseling, coaching, and "playshops" for adults. She also teaches at the University of Northern Iowa for the Department of Educational Leadership, Counseling, and Postsecondary Education. Terry developed Adlerian play therapy, an approach to counseling children that combines the ideas and techniques of Individual Psychology and play therapy. She is the author of *Partners in Play: An Adlerian Approach to Play Therapy* (1st and 2nd editions), *Play Therapy: Basics and Beyond*, and several other books on play therapy and counseling children. Most importantly, she is Jacob's mother and Rick's wife.

Donald DeGraaf, PhD, CTRS, is professor and chair of the Physical Education and Recreation Department at Calvin College. He has written and presented in the areas of camping, environmental ethics, adventure education, and the management of leisure service organizations. Don is the coauthor of *Camps and Youth Serving Programs: A Staff Development Approach* (with R. Ramsing, J. Gassman, and K. DeGraaf), *Programming for Parks, Recreation, and Leisure Service Organizations: A Servant Leadership Approach* (with D. Jordan and K. DeGraaf), and *Leisure and Life Satisfaction: Foundational Perspectives* (1st and 2nd editions; with C. Edgington, D. Jordan, and S. Edgington). Don and his wife Kathy live in Grand Rapids, Michigan, with their two children, Isaac and Rochelle.

Together, Jeff, Terry, and Don have presented at conferences, written articles, and taught a variety of classes and workshops pertaining to developing and facilitating adventure education–therapy programs. In 2001, they coauthored *Adventures in Guidance*, also published by the American Counseling Association. Together, and individually, Jeff, Terry, and Don have presented and trained in adventure activities in Asia, Europe, Africa, and all over the United States.

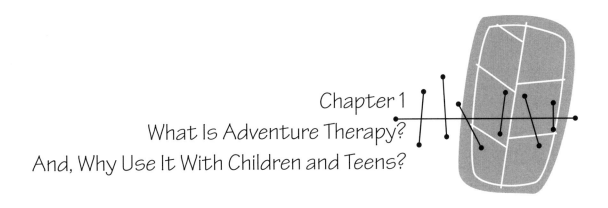

Chapter 1
What Is Adventure Therapy?
And, Why Use It With Children and Teens?

When the clinician uses a playful therapy style, the child not only gets great benefit from the message that he [or she] is a fun kid to be with, but also learns play-skills that often need to be part of the treatment plan.

—Beverly James

In this chapter we'd like to try to ask and answer several questions. These include, What exactly is adventure therapy? Why use adventure therapy intervention strategies with children and teens? What do kids get out of it? Does it work? How do you use it in schools and in mental health settings? And importantly, What does it look like? For us, these are not just hypothetical or academic questions. We regularly use these activities, and so it is not unusual for us to be asked questions like this in a sort of "What in the world are you doing?" tone of voice. You can imagine this also as you think about treating children or adolescents and explaining to their parents that in your last group session with their child/youth you played Bump (p. 49). It seems reasonable that you might get the direct question, "And why did you do *that* in session?" or the raise of the eyebrow, nonverbally communicating the same thing. In the age of empirically supported treatments and research support for interventions (both in mental health settings and in schools), we are sometimes asked if we ever use any interventions with any research support, rather than just playing games. We are also often queried about when the "real" therapy or counseling starts, assuming that the games will end soon because they can't be part of the intervention. If these kinds of questions don't sound familiar, they might be coming your way soon (especially if you start having FUN using this book). The sections that follow explore the ways we typically respond to these types of questions and then consider what adventure therapy looks like.

What Exactly IS Adventure Therapy?

There are probably lots of different definitions for adventure therapy, but hey, it's our book, so we'll offer ours. We describe adventure therapy as the use of games, activities, initiatives, and peak experiences to facilitate the development of group process, interpersonal relationships, personal growth, and therapeutic gain. Adventure therapy is an experiential therapy. Although there is an important processing (e.g., sit or stand around and talk about things) component to many adventure therapy activities, the main emphasis is on the experience of the activity. Hattie, Marsh, Neill, and Richards (1997) noted that, "The most striking common denominator of adventure programs is that they involve doing physically active things away from the person's normal environment" (p. 44).

Why Use Adventure Therapy Intervention Strategies With Children and Teens?

We often respond to this question with a question of our own: "Have you tried getting a group of preadolescent boys to sit quietly and talk productively for 50 full minutes? How's that gone for you?" (Because we have, and it hasn't really gone that well for us). This is perhaps a bit harsh, but it does speak to the point. One main reason for using these strategies is that children and teens want to MOVE.

(We actually think that adults want to move also—but that is for a different book.) In our experience, most parents, teachers, and other counselors have talked and talked and talked to these children and teens, often with minimal success. We're not against talking. In fact, we have "processing questions" for all of the activities in which we try to set you up for success in talking about the activities (in a way that moves toward accomplishing specific goals and objectives). Our main point is that participating in experiential interventions (like the 50 outlined in chapter 7) gives children and teens a chance to move and to "experience" some of the things we'd like them to think about and realize, rather than simply talking about them. For instance, we have found significant value in engaging children and teens in activities in which they can practice applying decision-making skills to resolve conflicts (see Goal 3, Objective F in Appendix A), get feedback about their behavior, and practice again in a different, though equally novel, setting. Although it is great to talk about conflict resolution and decision making, and even to role-play these (which offers the opportunity for feedback), it has been invaluable for us to have children and teens engage in activities (that don't feel like role-plays) in which these skills can be practiced and modeled and in which the "logical consequences" of not applying decision-making skills to resolve conflicts are felt.

This example rings true for us for nearly all of these goals and objectives (see Appendix A). If we have had the chance to do an activity that points to a specific goal and objective, we have a shared experience to which we can make reference. Teens often say, "It's just like when we played _____" when the "_____" is an activity in which the issues being discussed were represented in the activity. When the activity is fun and not too intense, it becomes an emotionally safer point of reference to talk about (as in our earlier conflict resolution and decision-making example, compared to a real conflict with parents, teachers, siblings, or other authority figures).

Another reason for using these activities, though we tend not to lead with it in discussions but is nonetheless important to us, is that children and teens have fun with these activities. We want clients to participate in therapy. We find that the likelihood for them to be open and engage in therapy is enhanced when they are having fun. Many of the activities are intentionally designed to be fun.

What Do Kids Get Out of It?

This is a slightly different question than the preceding one, though the answer has some overlap. What we often find is that the question "What do kids get out it?" is really a question of "If this stuff (adventure games and activities) works, why or how does it work?" We've written a little about this in other places (e.g., Kottman, Ashby, & DeGraaf, 2001), but we want to give a quick review and expansion. In brief, we think that when children and teens participate in these activities, led carefully, set up well, and processed intentionally, that positive change can occur. How? Ah, there's the rub…

When children and teens participate in these types of activities, it is likely that they will get enhanced self-efficacy (Bandura, 1986). You may recall that self-efficacy is the expectation or belief that one can accomplish a certain task or set of tasks. You may also recall that, in certain domains, self-efficacy is a better predictor of performance than ability. Simply put, low self-efficacy handicaps children and teens, socially and academically. Self-efficacy is related to a variety of other measures of well-being like self-esteem (see Bandura, 1986, for an extensive review). Adventure activities give children and teens the opportunity to enhance self-efficacy through the three primary sources of self-efficacy: performance accomplishments, vicarious learning, and verbal persuasion. If through participation in these activities, children and teens can accomplish tasks, see others accomplish tasks (in both cases including using skills, interpersonal strategies, impulse control, etc.), and get feedback about their actions and attitudes during the activities, self-efficacy generalized to other domains can be enhanced. A very good thing.

One can also frame the value of adventure activities from a client-centered perspective (Rogers, 1959). Consistent with the explanatory therapeutic factors of client-centered therapy, adventure activities allow participants to freely express their feelings, test reality, and become more discerning in their perceptions of the environment, self, others, and experiences. The activities allow participants a structured way to test self-perceptions in a context of trust and acceptance (facilitated by the group activities).

Another great answer to the question is based on Yalom's (1985) primary factors of a therapeutic experience. Yalom contended that group therapy "worked" for a number of reasons that included the instillation of hope ("I can get better"), universality ("other people feel the way I do"), the imparting of information ("I can learn from others"), altruism ("I care about others"), the corrective recapitulation of the primary family group ("I can re-experience early family experiences in potentially better ways"), development of socializing techniques ("I can connect with others"), interpersonal learning ("I can learn from interacting with you"), and group cohesiveness ("I'm a part of something"). Adventure therapy activities offer a somewhat unique platform for each of these therapeutic factors. When children and teens try to solve a problem together, after building some sense of group cohesion, they emphatically feel a part of something (group cohesion). As they work through the complex interpersonal dynamics of solving a problem under stress, they learn from interacting with each other (interpersonal learning and developing socializing techniques). They are likely to feel a sense of shared experience that the group is in it together (universality). Although Yalom argued for these factors being present, and curative, in traditional group psychotherapy, we are convinced that they may be even more evident, and just as curative, in groups using adventure challenge activities. It stands to reason that these would be felt with more salience when a group has come together and is working together to solve a problem or meet a challenge than they would from sitting in the room together as you do in traditional group psychotherapy.

Further, and as you can probably tell from our discussion thus far, we think of adventure techniques as techniques that can be conceptualized and explained from a variety of theoretical perspectives. If you are a Cognitive Behaviorist, we think adventure therapy techniques can help your clients shift their schemas and illuminate cognitive distortions in addition to allowing a context for behavioral practice for new ways of acting in the world (e.g., Beck, 1976). If you are a Gestalt therapist, we think that adventure therapy techniques can help your clients address unfinished business and work in the "here and now" of the activities (Yontef & Jacobs, 2005). If you are a contemporary psychodynamic therapist, we think that adventure techniques can offer your clients a unique environment to develop transference, come to insight, and develop intellectual and emotional mastery of previously unaddressed material (Arlow, 2005). If you're Adlerian, we think you can use adventure therapy techniques to build relationships with clients, help them explore their lifestyles, help them gain insight into their lifestyles, and learn and practice problem-solving and communication skills (Kottman, 2002). In short, we think that adventure techniques can be a valuable addition to your therapeutic toolkit no matter what your theoretical orientation.

This All Sounds Good—But Does It Really Work?

Ah yes, the understandable demand for empirical support. Although therapists might not like it, there is an increasing demand for empirical support for interventions. School systems need it, private practitioners need it, and mental health system workers need it. It is a reality of the millennium. So, to that end, we're happy to respond.

Does this stuff work? The easiest response is to reference the classic research article by Hattie et al. (1997). Hattie et al. conducted a meta-analysis based on 1,728 effect sizes drawn from 151 unique samples from 96 different studies. They found an average effect size of .34 with a follow-up effect size of .17. Hans (2000), in a more recent meta-analysis, found similar effect sizes. The outcomes measured in the included studies were a variety of self-concept, interpersonal, and personality variables. So children and adolescents who participated in these programs and/or received these interventions experienced a decrease in a variety of symptoms and an increase in well-being. In addition, the effect sizes are comparable to those found for individual psychotherapy (Wampold, 2001). In other words, YES. Of course there is also a great deal of anecdotal evidence regarding the efficacy of these techniques. Although, on the face of it, these stories and examples may not be scientifically compelling, we have found that they are a great way to illustrate and amplify the quantitative data provided by folks like Hattie et al. and Hans.

How Do I Use Adventure Activities at School?

We think that adventure activities are uniquely suited to a variety of school settings (Kottman et al., 2001). One prominent way that these activities are used is in classroom guidance. According to the American School Counselor Association (ASCA; 1984), developmental guidance is a program that "vigorously stimulates and actively facilitates the total development of individuals in all areas" (p. 1).

We are obviously biased, but still don't think you can find a better set of techniques than adventure therapy to "vigorously stimulate" and "actively facilitate" students' development. Because these activities can include, in many cases, up to 30 participants, they naturally lend themselves to classroom guidance situations. In addition, because the activities can be facilitated and processed to accomplish specific goals and objectives (see Appendix A), counselors can simply substitute these activities in the place of other targeted techniques or activities intended to accomplish a specific objective.

School counselors can also use these activities with groups they may be running. For instance, if a counselor is running a group for grief issues, social skills, divorce recovery, or some other focused topic, the counselor is likely to have specific goals for each of the group sessions. Counselors can use these activities to facilitate the group's development (e.g., cohesion, rapport, process) as well as to accomplish specific goals. Adventure activities can be a great way to shake up the group. Many school counselors use one activity a session, then use other techniques (e.g., art, discussion, role-play). Others use the adventure activities in several, but not all, of the planned group sessions. Further, school counselors can run an entire topic-focused group using exclusively adventure activities.

One other way school counselors use adventure activities is in one-on-one situations with clients. Any of the paired activities (that participants do with a partner) can be used in individual counseling (the pair in this case being you and the client). Using adventure therapy techniques with your individual clients is a way of bringing more experiential work into your counseling. Some clients respond to art and storytelling, but other clients may respond more to the active nature of these activities (think BOYS here—at least that has been our experience).

How Do I Use These Activities in Mental Health Settings?

Again, we're biased, but we think that adventure activities are a great match for mental health settings! One way we've used adventure activities is to facilitate learning in psychoeducational groups. Because the activities can be introduced, facilitated, and processed in a variety of ways to accomplish a variety of goals, they can be utilized to illustrate and begin discussion on a variety of psychoeducational topics. Another way we've used these activities in mental health settings is to do the activities with families. Some of the activities are suited to a single family unit (e.g., ideal with three to six participants), while others may be more suited to a family group (with more than one family in the group). We have found that using these activities with families can break down barriers and increase discussion. They provide a shared experience that can serve as a reference point for all family members in discussion. Adventure activities can also be a great diagnostic tool, as you can watch family members relate to each other (or not), trust each other (or not), and work to solve problems (again, or not).

Similar to the work of school counselors, adventure therapy techniques can be used in mental health group counseling settings. The activities can be used to facilitate group development (e.g., helping the group come together more quickly) as well as to lead to specific goals and objectives for the group counseling session. Especially with teens and children, we have found adventure activities a great way to accelerate group development. The adventure therapy components of active movement, some self-disclosure, laughter, and fun have proven extremely effective in our experience in helping group members get to know one another, relate to one another, and feel comfortable talking about a range of issues. We've found that this process can develop without adventure therapy techniques; it just develops faster with them!

Adventure activities can also be used in mental health group counseling settings to meet or address specific treatment plan goals. Again, as in school counseling settings, adventure activities can be explained, facilitated, and processed to accomplish specific goals for group sessions. We have found this particularly helpful when we were leading a topic-focused group (e.g., trauma, eating disorders) and had a specific goal for the group session.

Further, one other way counselors and therapists in mental health settings use adventure activities is in individual counseling. As noted earlier, therapists may choose do any of the paired activities (that participants do with a partner) in individual therapy (with the therapist and client being the pair). We have found the use of adventure activities with individual clients to be helpful with both children and teens. Children are used to play and may be familiar with play therapy interventions, and teens appreciate the chance to move and experience some of therapy rather than just talking.

What Does Adventure Therapy Look Like?

We've grouped the activities into four broad categories (with some overlap) based on the work of School and Maizell (2002). One way to think about these groups of activities is as a way to sequence activities to get to a particular goal or objective. That is, these activities can be used in isolation (e.g., a single trust activity) or as a bridge to other activities. Part of what we mean by *bridge* is that if we'd like a group to get to the working stage and have members give each other feedback, we may see Challenge/Initiatives as the best way to do that. However, it is hard to start with Challenge/Initiatives without sequencing up to them. The order of the activities presentation (Icebreaker, Deinhibitizer, Trust, Challenge/Initiative) is the sequence that School and Maizell suggested to gain optimal participation and usefulness from activities. We think if you'll read ahead you'll catch on quickly!

Icebreakers

Icebreakers are great beginning activities (because they break the ice). Icebreakers are designed to be fun, nonthreatening, and emphasize a success orientation. In Icebreakers, fun is a primary emphasis. Participants are often asked to be a little silly (though not TOO silly as that can be a little too challenging, especially if you don't know the other people in the group too well yet). Icebreakers may ask participants to make some small personal disclosure or put themselves in interpersonal situations with a minimum of personal risk (e.g., get up out of your chair, move around, toss a ball). It can be the first step in building relationships. As a result, Icebreakers are ideally nonthreatening. They are a way of inviting participants into a group setting by offering a chance to learn a little about the other participants and share an experience that is fun. Some group process can develop as the group laughs, moves, and shares. Icebreakers are not designed to be competitive (that can come later!), so there is little pressure to win or succeed. One primary objective of Icebreakers is to provide opportunities for participants to get to know the therapist. We often think of Icebreakers as techniques to facilitate the therapeutic alliance between client and therapist. Gelso and Carter (1985) noted that the working alliance includes a sense of trust between client and therapist and a sense of shared goals. One of the distinctions of Icebreakers is that the leader often gets to participate. This participation in a fun activity can build a sense of trust and lets clients see you as a fun person who is not threatening. As a result, we think clients are more likely to share more openly more quickly. In addition, Icebreakers allow the therapist the opportunity to gather diagnostic information. We use the word *diagnostic* in the broadest sense. As we see clients participate in Icebreakers, we are gathering information about how clients are relating to each other, how verbal they are, how generally cooperative, how rambunctious, how self-aware, and a variety of other variables. This information helps us formulate treatment plans and design interventions (both adventure activities and other types of interventions) that might best fit the group. A simple example is to do an initial Icebreaker with a group and note that, for whatever reason, the group is very active, you might even say WILD, today. As a result, we might choose a different next activity (say one that does not involve ball tossing that, with the group's current demeanor, might quickly turn into a violent dodge-ball scenario we did NOT plan on and that could undermine any positive group development).

Although Icebreakers are great beginning activities that can provide a bridge to other activities, they can also be processed metaphorically. In chapter 4 we talk a lot about processing and using metaphors (we won't steal that thunder at this point). Icebreakers are great beginning activities. They can help with the development of group process and the therapeutic alliance. They are great bridge activities that can set up other, potentially more challenging, interpersonally risky, or competitive activities. They can serve as assessment activities that give you helpful information about what kind of group it is or the current disposition of the group. Icebreakers can also be stand-alone activities that can be processed effectively and lead to discussions and learning that accomplish your goals and objectives (all while having some fun!).

Deinhibitizers

Deinhibitizers are activities we use when the group has developed a little bit of process. It is helpful if participants know each other's names. (Icebreakers don't necessarily require this and often facilitate it.) Although Icebreakers are activities that seem natural with brand new groups, Deinhibitizers might seem more of a stretch with new groups. They invite participants to be a little more vulnerable or exposed with the people in the group. As a result, if you began a group with a Deinhibitizer, some might opt out because they were uncomfortable with the level of silliness or potential embarrassment with folks they don't know very well. (This may also be personality driven. On a continuum, Jeff would likely be the most prone to choosing not to participate, while Terry would probably be game, although this is also situational.) However, when Deinhibitizers follow Icebreakers we find that the stretch is not so great because some initial group process is likely to have developed during the Icebreaker (e.g., knowing others' names).

One of the distinctives of Deinhibitizers is that they can be extremely SILLY. (Think silly in a good way.) They emphasize fun and good effort over success or failure in the activity. Deinhibitizers are typically designed to provide opportunities for participants to take some small personal risks and increase commitment. These risks can include a slightly larger degree of self-disclosure and of showing a willingness to appear inept in front of others. Because the participants are all in the same boat disclosing and or trying things that they've never tried, and never really seen a need to try, Deinhibitizers can facilitate group development. This shared experience and initial trust building also facilitates the development of the therapeutic alliance. Participants may be asked to put themselves in more challenging or silly situations. Deinhibitizers reinforce a cooperative and supportive atmosphere that encourages participation and appropriate risk taking. They also provide a context for clients to practice taking some emotional and physical risks, with some possible minor discomfort and/or frustration (moving clients out of their comfort zones). Like Icebreakers, Deinhibitizers can be correctly conceptualized as important bridge activities (leading to other, potentially more intense activities) and assessment activities (a way to gather much salient information about the group and individuals). They can also, like Icebreakers, be effective stand-alone activities. They can be led and processed in a way that can lead to specific objectives and goals. However, as we mentioned earlier, we use Deinhibitizers with groups who have gotten to know each other a little and developed some amount of group process (i.e., had the ice broken) either through earlier Icebreaker activities or through other means.

Trust Activities

The nature of Trust activities is relatively self-evident—they involve trust. One specific objective of Trust exercises is to provide opportunities for participants to trust their physical and emotional safety to others. Trust activities generally include involvement and interaction, both physically and verbally. They allow participants the opportunity to allow others to trust them, and thus prove trustworthy, and to trust others, giving them the chance to prove trustworthy. This is generally done through physical trust (e.g., physical touch and support). In trust activities, participants can learn what it is like to have others lean (often literally) on them and find them trustworthy ("I let you physically lean on me, and I didn't drop you! You trusted me, and I came through for you."). Trust activities are fun, but can involve a small amount of fear as well. Trust activities also require the support and cooperation of group members in some instances to care for the safety of others. For these reasons, it is important to sequence up to Trust activities (e.g., using Icebreakers and Deinhibitizers). It would obviously be a risky proposition (in a variety of ways) to begin with Trust activities. We have found it helpful for people to know each other's names and have some level of comfort and familiarity before we ask them to take charge of the physical safety of others (which often happens in Trust activities) or let others take responsibility for their safety. Icebreakers and Deinhibitizers can develop the group process that make Trust activities a relatively comfortable next step.

Challenge/Initiative Activities

The last category we use for activities is Challenge/Initiative activities. The distinction of these activities is that they really draw on what groups may get from earlier activities (i.e., Icebreakers, Deinhibitizers, Trust activities). In Challenge/Initiative activities, there is typically a challenge, either a problem to solve or a task to accomplish. The task or problem is generally a group problem that will require participants to effectively communicate, cooperate, and compromise with one another. To that end, group members need to know each others' names, be comfortable with one another, have some level of trust, and have had practice communicating. As a group has formed and developed, that shared sense of the group can contribute to the motivation to accomplish the task or solve the problem. Challenge/Initiatives have the advantage of feeling stressful to participants. These stressful situations of problem solving and responding to a challenge have a great parallel to life. They give participants the chance to practice new behaviors, give each other feedback, and get some feedback about how they are perceived and what kind of changes they have made or could make. These activities highlight the importance of listening, cooperating, and compromising. Further, the other advantage is these things all happen in the context of FUN.

Conclusion

In this chapter we've tried to give you a quick introduction to adventure therapy, what it is, how it works, that it works, etc. We've tried to answer questions you might have and give you some potential responses to questions others might have. We've also given a quick overview of the categories of activities included in chapter 7. If you'd like to skip to those activities (if you haven't already perused them), you can go there now. However, we have several other chapters on designing and implementing adventure interventions, so if you're interested, read on!

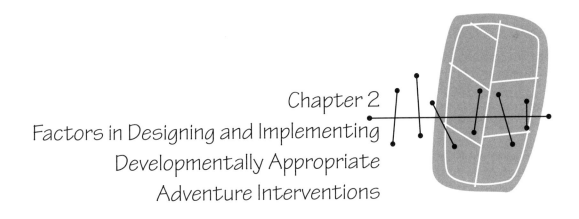

Chapter 2
Factors in Designing and Implementing Developmentally Appropriate Adventure Interventions

There are certain things that are important in thinking about working with children and adolescents when you are getting ready to do adventure activities (you are getting ready to do this, right?). What will work with one client might not work with another. (We know, that was obvious, but we needed to say it anyway.) So thinking things through before you even introduce the idea of adventure to the client(s) can make all the difference in whether you get the results you want (or not). In order to be able to design and implement developmentally appropriate adventure interventions with all of your clients, you need to consider their developmental levels. Obviously, you also need to consider individual clients and their particular likes and dislikes, wishes, and needs, because sometimes those factors will override the usual developmental factors. If you are using a group approach, in addition to the developmental considerations, you need to think about group composition, space considerations, level of trust present among the group members, and the purpose of the group. You also need to think about what you want to accomplish with that particular client (or group of clients) and whether adventure is the way to go. This is really the most important thing of all.

OK: What Does the Developmental Level of the Client Matter?

You already know this: Kids at different levels of development require handling tailored to that particular developmental level. What will work with a kindergarten kid often won't work in exactly the same way with a fifth grader. What will work with a sixth grader may not work with a senior in high school. Well, the basic activity will probably work (check those age ranges on the activity descriptions just to make sure), but you will need to adapt a number of things to ensure that the activity will work with particular populations. Just in general, younger children (e.g., early primary grades) require more specific instructions, detailed suggestions about how to organize themselves, less time on each activity, more supervision, more concrete processing, smaller groups (or subgroups), simpler vocabulary, and fewer processing questions. With older children (e.g., later elementary grades) and adolescents, you can generally get away with letting them figure out many aspects of the game themselves (like who goes first, how to divide into subgroups, what to do with sparse instructions), having bigger groups (or subgroups), and expecting more complex and abstract processing.

What Developmental Factors Do I Need to Consider in Working With the Various Age Groups?

We have (rather arbitrarily, we admit) divided child development into primary grade children, intermediate grade children, middle school/junior high school youth, and high school youth. This division makes sense to us, and we hope it does to you as well. For each developmental level, we have discussed some important factors in development, how each of the types of activities will work with that level, what to consider when thinking about whether to use an individual or group approach, what kinds of structuring are required for playing and processing, how long an adventurous session should last and how you might want to spend the time in the session, and how to think about the process of processing.

Primary Grade Children (Grades K, 1, and 2)

Primary grade children like to move, and they like to play (Muro & Kottman, 1995; Thompson & Henderson, 2006; Vernon, 2004; Vernon & Clemente, 2005), so adventure therapy techniques present an excellent intervention strategy to use with this age group. You just have to remember a couple of things to make sure that primary age children get the most they can out of your activities. Icebreakers and Deinhibitizers work really well with children this age: they love permission from a grown-up to move around and be silly. However, if they think they already know the rules to a game and you are asking them to play the game in a way different from how they think it should go, sometimes that is tricky. You may have to convince them that playing the game a new way can be even more fun than playing it the way they already know. Many primary grade children are willing to do trust activities because they have not learned to be distrustful. You will need to make sure that they take the task of keeping another person safe seriously and don't get too silly because this can result in problems in trust activities—like crashing someone into a wall or into another person. Challenge/Initiative activities can also work with this age children, but you will just need to keep the challenges reasonable because they do not have as many coping strategies as older children do to help them deal with the frustrations inherent in many of the Challenge/Initiative activities.

Both individual and group approaches work with primary age children. They like to do things with adults—especially adults who have already established a relationship with them, like their teacher, their counselor, or a staff member who regularly works with them—so an individual counseling relationship that includes adventure activities, along with other play therapy techniques (Kottman, 2001), can be very productive. Primary grade children also enjoy doing things in groups: they like each other and have decided (for the most part) that playing with other kids is just as good (sometimes even better) than that parallel play they did for so long. They haven't developed the idea that the members of the opposite sex have cooties yet, so activities that require hand-holding won't even be a problem.

Primary grade children need more structuring than older children. This means that you will need to be very specific and concrete in explaining the directions to your activities, so in activities in which our directions are purposely vague, you may need to adapt them to make sure children understand what is supposed to happen. That way you will avoid them spending all the time you have allotted to a particular activity answering questions. If you are doing a group and have subgroups, dyads, or triads, you will need to help children do the dividing—like counting off or specifying, "Find someone else whose name starts with the same letter as yours." You also need to help them figure out who has which role in the game (such as by saying things like, "OK: the person who is the shortest is It first."). With primary grade children, it is helpful to keep your group rather small or divide the larger group into subgroups, with an adult facilitator assigned to the subgroups when possible. (We know, that might be a luxury not found in the real world, but—) If you do have subgroups, you should keep them small, with only three or four in each subgroup. Also helpful is to have a greater adult–child ratio with these children, because it is helpful to have more supervision than you need with older children. If you are doing a group and the children's teacher, parent, or supervisor (like a cottage staff person in a residential setting or a floor staff in a hospital setting) is available to participate, sometimes this can help make the group more fruitful and the processing more meaningful because these adults are very important to children at this age.

You will want to keep the time you play with this age group relatively short, probably about 20 minutes (half hour at the most), because their attention spans are still relatively limited. Keeping the main emphasis on the playing of the activities and limiting your time spent processing will also be helpful. If we were going to use adventure techniques with a child (or a group of children) in Grades K–2, we would do an activity that lasted about 15 minutes and process for 5 (at the most).

Children at this level tend to be oriented to the here-and-now (Muro & Kottman, 1995; Vernon, 2004; Vernon & Clemente, 2005), so asking the personalization-processing questions will usually be more fruitful than the application-processing questions, which are often past- and future-oriented. While they are gradually starting to outgrow the egocentrism of early childhood, primary grade children still sometimes struggle with taking the cognitive and emotional perspectives of others, so asking them to consider what someone else thinks or feels about a situation is usually futile (and frustrating to you and them). Children at this age have not yet developed the ability to consider in an abstract way, so keeping your processing concrete seems to work better—asking things like, "What did you like best when we played this?" or "What was hard for you when we played this?" will work well. Another technique that works well with this age group is making guesses or sharing tentative hypotheses about what is going on with children, rather than asking them questions (Muro & Kottman, 1995; Thompson & Henderson, 2006). When you do this, you will need to watch for the *recognition reflex*, a nonverbal reaction that telegraphs clients' reactions to your guess, because children will not always respond verbally to guesses, even when they are accurate.

Intermediate Grade Children (Grades 3 Through 5/6)

Intermediate grade children (at least in our experience) are the perfect clients for adventure therapy strategies. They are aware of their feelings, and they are willing and able to talk about them. They have begun to develop the capacity for insight into themselves and into others, and they like to interact actively with other people, especially their peers (Muro & Kottman, 1995; Thompson & Henderson, 2006; Vernon, 2002, 2004; Vernon & Clemente, 2005). Most kids in this age range are willing to participate (and savor) all four of the types of activities. Icebreakers and Deinhibitizers are valued as a chance for sanctified silliness and movement. However, this age group does tend toward becoming self-conscious more easily than younger children, so at times they may struggle with the more outrageous deinhibitizing activities. (After all, so many things are potentially embarrassing to kids at this age.) They also don't always like to be the center of attention (especially fifth and sixth graders), so some of the storytelling techniques may not be their cup of tea. Intermediate grade children are still (for the most part) pretty trusting, so they are usually willing to participate in Trust activities. You need to be aware of which children might be the ones who push it—either do reckless things or might do something to endanger a partner. With the children who would be careless with their own safety or the safety of others, usually the proximity of a leader who is obviously monitoring their behavior or providing verbal reminders about safety or redirection toward safer behavior is usually enough to insure that there are no casualties. You also need to be aware of those individuals who have had experiences that make trusting someone else a difficult or painful process. With children who would find a Trust activity too stressful, it may be better to excuse them from a group trust process or pair them with an adult they know they can trust. Challenge/Initiative activities seem to be a favorite of intermediate grade children. They love to solve problems—the more complex the better. We tend to start with easier challenges to build up their sense of self-efficacy and ability to cooperate with others, and then move to more difficult challenges. At this age, most children have developed strategies for coping with stress and frustration, and they may still need reminders to apply those strategies during this type of activity.

Individual counseling works well with intermediate grade children, especially if you use active techniques such as adventure activities and art experiences, to engage them in the process because they might not want to sit around and just talk to a counselor or therapist. A group approach may work even better than individual counseling, especially with older children in this age range. As the peer group grows in importance, gradually replacing the influence of adults, other children and their inclusion and acceptance become the be-all and end-all for many children. They care about what other children think and feel about them, they care about finding their place in the group—and a group counseling approach can help with this.

The younger children in this age range have often come to believe that members of the opposite sex have cooties, and the older children in this age range have often started to be aware of their attraction (or attractiveness) to others, so activities that involve touching one another can be tricky. In order to avoid the "ewwww" reactions we sometimes get when we ask kids to hold hands during an activity, we often have them hold on to unrolled socks rather than one another. However, there are some activities, like Human Camera (p. 105) or Carry That Load (p. 52), that require more touching than just holding hands. You can decide whether to just not use these activities or to figure out a way to make the touching part something to process. We have observed that sometimes when there is a task to be accomplished (as in Carry That Load), the whole touching thing doesn't come up because the members of the group are so focused on solving the problem.

Intermediate grade children don't need as much structuring as primary grade children, but they still do need some structuring. You will need to give them directions (obviously), but the directions can be a little vague. We usually give the directions and then allow questions, and sometimes we even answer them. At this age, children often need some kind of guidance in deciding who goes first, who is It, or who is in which subgroup (if you are using them). Be creative in how you tell them to decide (first birthday, longest hair, shortest fingernails, highest jumper, fastest at solving a math problem, etc.). If you are playing an activity with teams, figure out a way for them to be divided without someone picking the members of the team. We usually use the number system, going around the circle counting off (1, 2, 1, 2, etc.) to decide who is on which team for activities. We tend to use pairs with this age group, or we have bigger subgroups than we did with younger children. Six or eight kids in a group seems to work really well, actually. With fewer kids than this, they don't seem to get that group feeling, and with more kids than this, not everyone gets to talk (VERY important with this age). It is also extremely helpful still to have an adult in the group (or in each subgroup) to lead the processing by, for example, calling on folks who want to talk, drawing out folks who are not so forthcoming, following up on answers that seem to need deepening, or making sure that just one or two kids don't monopolize the conversation. If you are using subgroups and you have the luxury of having adults assigned to subgroups, remind them that they are not to solve the problems for the children nor are they to do a lot of self-disclosure. In fact, the more invisible they are, the better: their job is to spotlight the kids, provide a little structuring, and keep things positive and encouraging.

With intermediate children, the time line is expanded. This age group has a much longer attention span and can do an hour or two at a time if your schedule allows for this. In fact, a longer session (lasting at least an hour and a half) that includes all four types of activities seems ideal for this age range. You can actually do an entire day of adventure activities. If you have a schedule that dictates shorter sessions (for example, if you are a school counselor doing classroom guidance, which usually lasts about a half hour, or a counselor or therapist in private practice who does 50-minute sessions), this will work too. You will just do fewer activities or confine what you are doing to a certain type of activity (remembering to sequence across sessions, rather than within sessions). We usually do an activity, then process that activity, then do another activity and process it. Children in this age range tend to require closure on a particular experience before they move on to the next experience, so doing several activities and then processing them together doesn't seem to work well. It is still important to have the activity–processing ratio weighted on the side of having more activities and fewer questions. We tend to play for 20 minutes to a half hour, then talk for 5 (maybe 10) minutes, then do another activity, and then talk some more.

There is a wide range of cognitive and affective abilities among intermediate grade children, so you will have to think about your particular clients as you consider how to adapt the processing. Some children in this age range are capable of abstract reasoning and deep personal insight, and others are not. With those children who are able, asking them the more complex questions about responsibility, personal boundaries, and cultural differences and stereotyping will help them to learn more about themselves and others. With other children who are more concrete, you may want to stay with the less abstract questions such as, "What did you like about this activity?" or "What did you learn from this activity?" or "What was stressful about this activity?" Even with children who are not interested in or capable of dealing with the more abstract probes, you can still ask questions like, "What was stressful about it?" or "What strategies did you use to cope with the stress?" Most children at this developmental level are capable of exploring both personalization-processing and application-processing questions. However, don't ask every single question we have listed for an activity: the number of questions you ask should be about one fourth to one half of the children's age (so with a 12-year-old child, three to six questions is good). With a group, ask fewer questions than you would with an individual child, so that everybody gets a chance to talk and everybody is still willing to listen. Also, pay attention to the nonverbals of the children: If they are bored or not into thinking about your questions, cut the processing and get to the playing. Sometimes less is more with the processing (and remember, we did say that you don't have to process verbally at all; just let the experience speak for itself).

Middle School/Junior High Youth

In middle school/junior high school, there is a bigger span of developmental levels than in any other time period (Cobb, 2001; Vernon, 2004; Vernon & Clemente, 2005). At times they will act in very adult ways, and at times it is as if they are still in preschool. Sometimes it seems as though the only predictable thing about this age group is their unpredictability. They are alternately insightful and sensitive and obtuse and callous. They may be willing to be vulnerable one minute and sprout defenses like a fortified castle the next. They may be the world's most talkative kids in one session and sullenly silent in the next. The main thing to remember with this age group is to deal with the kids you have at the moment, rather than being attached to them acting in a certain, preordained way.

All of the types of activities will work with this age group. They may be a bit leery of the Deinhibitizers because of the potential for embarrassment, and they may be leery of the Trust activities because of their own personal experiences with situations that require trust. Sequencing is extra important with this age group because they have such inherent difficulties with taking risks: they take too many, and they take too few. Youth in this developmental stage are often attracted to taking behavioral risks, while at the same time they may be especially reluctant to take emotional and interpersonal risks. Middle school/junior high school children tend to be more emotionally volatile than elementary age children, and this can affect their reactions to the Challenge/Initiative activities. Sometimes they get so frustrated with the process of trying to solve the problems in these activities (especially when the leader changes the rules on them or won't clarify the instructions), they have emotional outbursts or refuse to continue. This is unsettling, but it can be grist for your processing mill: generally, if a person has a strong emotional reaction during these activities, he or she is probably having similar emotional reactions in other situations and relationships. And sometimes feedback from a supportive group or an encouraging adult can be used as a teachable moment that might reduce future outbursts or meltdowns.

The general wisdom is that the way to go in counseling adolescents is the group approach. Group counseling is particularly appropriate for adolescents. Being in a group gives adolescents a place to express conflicting feelings, explore self-doubts, and come to the realization that they share these concerns with their peers (Corey, 2007; Gladding, 2002). In groups, younger adolescents can explore their values, learn to communicate with peers, safely explore limits, and contribute to the welfare of others. An adventure group is particularly well suited to this age range because it also encourages them to express themselves physically as well as verbally, and creates a safe space for them to experiment with risk taking (especially psychological and relational risks). However, particularly in the area of trust, there are times when an individual approach would be more appropriate. With those youth who struggle with connecting with others, building a trusting, encouraging relationship with an adult can be a preface to learning to connect with other adolescents. Doing individual sessions of adventure techniques might be the best avenue with these individuals.

This will come as no surprise, but middle school/junior high youth need considerably smaller amounts of structure than elementary students. With this developmental level, you can be just as vague as you want while explaining the activity. We are more likely to simply repeat the directions, rather than answering a lot of detailed questions, under the assumption that this age level can (and should) figure things out for themselves. Although we still avoid the picking of teams, we usually allow children in this age group to choose their own partners, choose who is going to be It first, or decide whether they want to use props for processing. We may also give them a choice of two different activities (though we choose the choices). With this age group, you can have a bigger group (or subgroups, with 10 or 12 people in each), though smaller groups (or subgroups) still have the greater likelihood that everyone who wants to talk gets to talk (and keeps those who don't want to talk from effectively hiding). It is still helpful, but not necessary, to have an adult in the group (or subgroups) to help facilitate processing.

Middle school/junior high students have a wide range of attention spans, so you will need to take your particular client population into account when thinking about how long a session should last and how to spend the time. For the most part, you can get away with a longer session than you could at the elementary level, usually between an hour and an hour and a half or even 2 hours. However, if you are doing an activity that is especially emotionally volatile or if you have an especially emotionally volatile group, you might want to keep your session to an hour or less. With this developmental level, you can divide your time equally between doing and talking—with half of your session devoted to the activities and the other half devoted to processing.

One of the biggest developmental considerations in working with adolescents is their shift from concrete to formal operational thinking (Kaplan, 2000; Schave & Schave, 1989; Vernon, 2004). This change starts at around age 11, but is not completed until sometime between ages 15 to 20 (Kaplan, 2000). Because of the uncertainty of when this shift occurs, there is an infinite variety of processing abilities in this age range. When formal operational thinking kicks in, individuals can detect inconsistencies, think about future changes, see possibilities, and think logically about decision making and problem solving (Vernon, 2004). Before this occurs, they may not be able to do these things, or if they can, they may not be able to apply these skills consistently. So depending on where individual adolescents are in this cognitive developmental process, they may revel in thinking about processing questions, or they may assiduously try to avoid thinking about much of anything but the hormones coursing through their bodies. (Sorry, maybe a little graphic, but the three of us all live with kids who are in this particular age group, and . . . you get the idea.) To a certain extent, deciding how much to process, what kinds of things to process, and how deep you go in the processing, is a trial-and-error situation with early adolescents. We ask some questions, see what happens, and then decide what kinds of additional questions to ask (or what kinds of answers to expect) and sometimes whether or not to ask any more questions at all.

High School Youth

By high school, adolescents exhibit many characteristics of adulthood. They have matured enough to be able to think abstractly, to consider the past and how it has formed them and to consider the future and what it holds for them. Adolescents at this age are very interested in "achieving independence and finding their identities—discovering who they are and are not" (Vernon, 2004, p. 25). They are very interested in clarifying their beliefs and values and exploring their relationships and responsibilities (well, sometimes). The majority of individuals at this developmental level have problem-solving and decision-making skills, but they still need practice in effectively solving problems and making appropriate decisions. They are capable of expressing their thoughts and feeling verbally, rather than having to act them out through their behaviors (Vernon & Clemente, 2005).

And most of them still like to have fun, so all of the types of activities can be used with this age group. If you are working with a group with members who don't know one another, it would be important to start with Icebreakers so that the members of the group learn names and have a vehicle for beginning to know one another. Many high school youth have developed a rather extensive set of inhibitions, especially related to physicality, so doing Deinhibitizers will help to loosen them up and deepen their relationships with one another. Trust tends to be an issue for many adolescents, so Trust activities will be important in helping them explore these issues and in fostering increased trust of self and others. Challenge/Initiative activities work well because they provide opportunities for applying problem-solving and decision-making skills, taking responsibility, exploring boundaries, expressing thoughts and feelings, enhancing positive attitudes and skills related to learning, and gaining insight into self and others.

In thinking about whether to use a group or individual approach, the common wisdom (Corey, 2007; Gladding, 2002) is that group counseling is the ideal intervention for working with adolescents. An adventure therapy group can provide a living laboratory for the members to experiment with improving communication skills, building relationships, increasing self-awareness and self-acceptance, cooperating with others, learning to understand and value diversity, and being consistently responsible. That being said, there are some adolescents who are just not comfortable in a group and others who are not yet ready for being in a group. You will have a good sense of the clients you work with and which ones are good candidates for including in a group and which ones would work better just with you.

If you are going to do a group with high school youth, you probably need to think about age and gender issues. According to Gladding (2002), high school freshmen and sophomores should not be put in a group with juniors and seniors, as their concerns are so different. There are arguments for and against mixed-gender groups at this age (Gladding, 2002). Sometimes sexual tension can make coed group interaction stressful and/or awkward. Adolescent females tend to be more at ease with sharing their feelings than adolescent males, and this may make mixed-gender groups rather lopsided. However, the value of a coed group is that the boys can learn from the girls and vice versa. Your own personal comfort level and your setting may dictate whether you choose to mix girls and boys in a group.

Just as with middle school/junior high school youth, high school youth generally need limited forms of structuring. You can be very vague in your directions, letting them figure out how to do what they need to do. Jeff and Don love simply to repeat the original directions over and over again. Terry, who is more of a pleaser, tends to try to clarify stuff and usually makes things worse. So do whatever works for you in this area, but remember, they don't really need you to do this for them. (And they like to practice that independence—over and over and over again—so this is your chance to let them, even if the process is frustrating for them.) High school age clients can also generally figure out how to divide into dyads or subgroups, who is It first, how to start an activity, who should go first, and so forth, without any assistance from you. Sometimes we even let them pick their own teams.

With this age, because of their increased autonomy, you can definitely go for larger group (or subgroup) size if you want: 10 to 12 people will work nicely. However, if you want the members to go deeper with one another in the processing, you might want to consider a smaller group of six to eight. If you are using subgroups, you really no longer need an adult to facilitate interaction (unless you have behavioral concerns about the particular population in the group). It helps to have a leader of the big group who poses the processing questions, but you can easily count on the kids to monitor their own interaction, making sure that they all get a chance to contribute to the discussion. Many times they can even generate their own questions; and lots of times the questions they ask one another are better than anything any of us could think of. Depending on the quality of the interaction among your group members, you may be able to let them lead most of the processing. If you decide to do this, at the beginning of your time with them you want to model the kinds of questions you would usually ask and then gradually take yourself out of this role.

Like older elementary children and middle school/junior high school youth, older adolescents can tolerate and benefit from longer sessions than younger children. Because they usually have longer attention spans and interest, you can easily have a session that lasts an hour or two. With this population, if you have a setting that allows it, having adolescents play together for an entire day (or several days) also works very well. Depending on the individual or group (the folks who are in it and what you are trying to accomplish with them), you can choose to emphasize processing more than playing or you can choose to emphasize more playing than processing. With this age group, you can have them process a very long time, and some groups want to do just that. However, remember that the playing is always the catalyst for the talking, so don't neglect the playing even with the most talkative group.

With adolescents, the most important factor in thinking about how many and what kind of processing questions to ask is the particular goal for the counseling process. Individuals in this age group are able to consider and articulate their thoughts and feelings about a variety of topics. They are capable of self-examination at a deeper level than most younger clients are. So go for it! The sky is the limit: ask as many questions as you want about any subject you want. Just remember to think about whether your priority is the depth of the processing or the quantity of questions answered.

If I Am Doing a Group, What About Group Composition, Space Considerations, Level of Trust Present Among the Group Members, and the Purpose of the Group?

Many of these factors may not be in your control. In lots of these situations, someone else may have decided on group size, group purpose, and group composition (for example, if you are a school counselor and the principal says, "You need to do a friendship skills group with those 10 fourth-grade boys with ADHD"). You may work in a setting with no chance to influence who is in the group and how big it is (for example, if you work in residential treatment for adolescent sex offenders, you probably have to do group with whoever lives in a certain cottage). You may be working with an ongoing group that has been established for a while. You may be doing a one-shot group composed of the people who show up.

If you do have control of these factors (or at least have some way to influence them), here are some things to consider:

1. Generally, it is helpful to have some model children in your group. If you are working on social skills, it works better to have some participants in the group who actually have reasonable social skills, rather than having a bunch of participants who are learning new inappropriate social skills from one another.
2. Doing a group takes more space than working individually with clients. Adventure interventions take even more space than a normal group because of all that running around. You will need more than just a space that will accommodate a small circle of chairs.

3. Generally speaking, doing a group will require you to deliberately set things up to build trust among the members. Although this (hopefully) automatically happens between a counselor and the client in individual counseling, with a group there are many more people involved, all of whom need to have some level of trust in one another in order for a group to facilitate healing. You will need to monitor this closely and may need to create ways to use adventure activities (or art experiences or other counseling techniques) to help the level of trust in the group develop.

4. There are lots of different kinds of groups: personal growth groups, psychoeducational groups, topic-focused groups, or groups focused on specific problems or populations. The kind of group you are leading (and, again, your setting) will dictate, to a certain extent, what your purpose in the group will be. We believe that you should be very specific with yourself and with the members of the group about what you are trying to accomplish through the group process.

What Do I Want to Accomplish With This Client or Group of Clients?

Having goals and objectives to guide your interventions with clients makes the process more effica-cious and efficient (ASCA, 2005; Jongsma, Peterson, & McInnis, 2002, 2006). Thinking about what you want to accomplish (both short term and long term) can be extremely helpful in planning interven-tions with clients. Your setting may dictate the specific goals and objectives that you must include in your treatment plan, so you may not need any help with this. However, we have observed that many settings (both school and mental health work environments) provide limited guidance in this area. So we decided to include a list of goals and objectives that are appropriate for children and adolescents across the span of development. We believe the activities in this book can be instrumental in promot-ing client growth in these areas. We based these goals and objectives on our experience with children and adolescents, on consultation with school counselors and mental health providers who work with children and youth, on the ASCA national model for school counseling programs (ASCA, 2005), and on several guides used to help mental health practitioners develop treatment plans for children and adolescents (Jongsma et al., 2002, 2006). For each of the activities (in chapter 7), we have provided a number of goals and objectives we think you can accomplish using that particular activity. We don't want to limit you to using the activities just to accomplish those specific goals, however. We know there are lots of others: Use your imagination; go wild!

Chapter 3
How to Lead an Adventurous and Safe Group

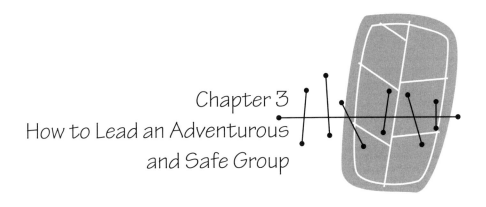

A group of tourists were visiting a village. As they walked by an old man sitting on a fence, one of the tourists asked, "Were there any great men or women born in this village?" The old man replied, "No, only babies."
—*Viata Training Manual* (2005, p. 7)

A casual observer watching a group engaged in the activity Protect the Jewels (p. 148) might see a simple game with participants attempting to physically steal "the good stuff" from one participant who is trying to protect it. Although it is true that the participants are having fun, if done well (as we're sure you will), the activity is much more than a fun game. If the observer sticks around long enough, he or she might see the group discuss what makes up the good stuff in their classroom, family, or personal lives and the kinds of things that can steal the good stuff. In addition, the members of the group might discuss how they can work together and even recruit others to protect that good stuff. The activity can be a powerful tool for developing a safe environment for participants, both individually and as a group. It creates a context for learning, insight, and transfer, and helps the group members identify what they are going to pay attention to while they are together. It becomes a visual metaphor for the group members about how they can work together to create the kind of family, classroom, or personal lives they want to achieve.

For us, this example illustrates the deceptive appearance of adventure activities and highlights that they are more than simply playing fun games (Frank, 2001). Adventure activities are an intentional attempt to facilitate specific treatment goals and objectives and enhance the clients' insight and learning. An integral part of the success of adventure activities is the counselor or therapist and the leadership skills he or she possesses. With this in mind, this chapter examines how to successfully lead the kind of activities described in chapter 7.

A good bit of the success of adventure activities has to do with how they are led. Successful leadership plays a significant role in determining whether the activity is really an intentional intervention that leads to the facilitation of treatment objectives. This kind of leading may also be outside of the normal skill set of counselors or therapists. (We never received this training!) So can you do it? We think you can guess our answer, but we'd also like to refer you back to the quote at the beginning of this chapter. The quote gives some insight into the age-old question, Are leaders born or made?

We believe that developing leadership skills is a never-ending learning process—starting with learning the leadership tools, techniques, and people skills needed to lead. We don't know any true born leaders, only babies who've grown into being GREAT at leading and processing adventure activities. As counselors and therapists gain experience in applying basic leadership techniques, they develop the confidence and ability to shape their leadership style to the demands of a given situation. In this way, leading activities can be seen as part art and part science. The art of leadership includes the intangible qualities of leadership that are critical to success, such as using sound judgment, integrating one's personality into activity leadership, and having a positive and upbeat attitude. These leadership elements are difficult to teach and are acquired and internalized over time. The science aspect of activity leadership can be taught and learned. It involves certain steps and much planning. This chapter focuses on the fundamentals of good leadership, and also gives you a variety of tools and techniques that you can use in leading adventure-based activities. Let's get started!

What Are the Fundamentals of Leading Adventure-Based Activities?

If you forget everything else in this entire chapter, remember that the most important factors in leading adventure-based activities are monitoring safety considerations, being intentional in using activities, showing enthusiasm, and having fun.

Safety

We list safety first because it is the most important element of leading adventure activities. Although at one level this goes without saying, we're saying it because it is a paradigm shift for most counselors and therapists to think about physical safety in addition to emotional or psychological safety. You are likely to be in tune with any kind of group work that might put participants at some level of emotional risk, but attending to physical risk is typically not a part of our mindset in traditional counseling and therapy settings. The paradigm shift includes, for us, thinking like a parent or a gym teacher (not sure if either of these come naturally to you). For example, we often think, in anticipating safety concerns, if our children were going to get hurt (as ours are prone to do), how could it happen in this activity?

In thinking about physical safety, we consider the participants, the setting, the activity itself, and the situation. For instance, is the activity a moving activity? If so, can people run into each other? Trip and fall? Run into obstacles (e.g., chairs, walls, desks, trees)? What is the space like? Will the space enhance the possibility of participants running into each other because, for example, it is a small space or because there are obstacles like chairs, desks, trees, etc.? If you are outside, what is the terrain? Are there curbs, concrete, grass, bushes, or traffic? Are there any inherent risks in the activity? Remember that any activity that involves touching another participant is potentially risky. From tagging to physically supporting participants, physical touch includes some potential risk. We have found that some of our participants can be fairly aggressive or have poor impulse control (hence their need for counseling). You can immediately think of potential safety concerns for any activity involving competition or projectiles (e.g., the idea is to gently toss the ball, but given aggressiveness and poor impulse control, a fairly violent and rather ugly spontaneous game of dodge ball can develop instead).

Once you are aware of any potential safety issues, the next step is working with the group to manage those hazards and to protect participants. It is important to remember that activity selection, sequencing, anticipation, planning, and empowerment all become tools for leaders in managing safety for individuals and groups throughout adventure experiences (Michaelis & O'Connell, 2000). To further assist you, we have included several techniques for monitoring safety during a group activity later in this chapter.

In addition to physical safety, good leaders (like you!) are also concerned about emotional and psychological safety. We have found that these concerns are much more on the radar of counselors and therapists than physical safety concerns typically are (based in large part on our previous training). However, one of the things that tends to slip by us is that many adventure activities are evocative. That is, they tend to raise issues for clients, sometimes in ways we hadn't expected. We recall the definition of adventure activities by Hattie et al. (1997) as doing physically active things in novel environments as we also recall that we have found that the new setting and novelty of activity tends to evoke reactions from clients. This is generally GREAT! We don't want the activities to be benign. We always hope to prompt discussion, etc. However, putting children and youth in these new contexts also can bring up issues sooner than they typically would arise in traditional counseling settings. We encourage you to keep this in mind and be prepared for the possibility of clients disclosing at a deeper level more quickly than they might in other settings, and perhaps more quickly than you had anticipated. We want to make sure that we have enough group process to support folks who make these disclosures.

Another emotional/psychological safety concern is that the group might turn on one or more participants. Because adventure activities are potentially stressful, and because participants don't always exhibit their most charitable behavior (e.g., name-calling, ganging up on a participant for his or her performance) under stress, there is the possibility of participants undermining the counseling process and even hurting others. Although this is always the case in group work, as you know, it is accentuated in adventure activities. Later in the chapter we talk about a variety of ways (e.g., setting the ground rules with participants) to anticipate emotional/psychological safety concerns.

Intentionality

As one of our favorite quotes states, "The secret of knowing how is remembering why." So in answering the question of how we lead adventure-based activities, the best place to start is by asking why we are using a specific activity. For what purpose are we choosing this specific activity over all other possible activities (like the other 49 in this book)? The Protect the Jewels (p. 148) example described at the beginning of the chapter is one example of how a leader can intentionally structure an experience to meet a specific treatment objective. The important point here is that we must plan what activities we use with great care, and be intentional about the outcome we want to produce.

The first step in leading adventure-based activities is to identify the *why*; once we have done this it allows us to begin with the end in mind. Much as an architect begins building a new structure with the help of blueprints, we begin building our programs when we know where we want to go and why we want to get there. Laying this foundation allows us to be intentional about how we get there by picking the right activity for the right group at the right time.

Enthusiasm and Passion

Enthusiasm is derived from the Greek word *en theos*, meaning "the spirit of god within" (those Greeks had a way with words, didn't they?). In terms of adventure activity leadership, enthusiasm is the personal spirit you as a leader contribute to the experience. Through enthusiasm, leaders can ignite the passion of others and get them excited about what they are doing. Enthusiastic leaders invite others into the play process, thereby encouraging participants to build a collective group enthusiasm. It's important to remember that each person's way of expressing his or her enthusiasm is a reflection of personal style. Some people may be loud and boisterous, others may be quiet with a spark of subtle humor. What is most important about enthusiasm is that it is genuine and from the heart (Michaelis & O'Connell, 2000).

We have found that enthusiasm is one of the best predictors of success in leading an adventure activity. If you can communicate your energy and excitement about the activity, this is contagious. Enthusiasm is the catalyst that enables participants to join fully in the activity and experience and to lose their self-consciousness about how silly or contrived the activity might have seemed to some of them initially. Enthusiasm helps participants engage more fully in the activity and, as a result, profit more from it.

Fun

We've already tried to be clear about our commitment to fun (see the Preface). One of the unique aspects of adventure-based activities is that they are experiential, which opens the possibility to make insight, growth, and learning active and fun. Sometimes in our efforts to lead effectively (safely, intentionally, enthusiastically), we can lose track of FUN. Successful leaders don't forget the fun. One way to do this is by developing a sense of playfulness (when appropriate) in our leading. This sense of playfulness will often flow out of our enthusiasm and passion for the activities we are leading. As a result, we want to be intentional and facilitate growth, and in the process, we want to remind you not to forget to be open to the opportunities to use humor and play to create a fun learning environment for our participants. One way we do this is by modeling FUN through participating in activities (e.g., Paint Your Name, p. 137) and having fun doing it.

What Do I Need To Do Before I Meet My Group?

Key to leading a successful adventure activity is planning and preparation. As we have already noted, being intentional about the purpose of an activity or program is extremely important. Once you have identified the purpose, you can begin to ask purpose-related questions, and get ready to formulate your plan.

Asking Purpose-Related Questions

Questions that need to be asked as you plan and prepare an adventure activity include

- *What are the developmental needs of your participants?* As highlighted in chapter 2, the developmental level of the participants makes a difference in a variety of adventure activity areas. In leading, you may want to consider issues of structure (e.g., primary grade children may need more structure than middle schoolers), complexity (e.g., high school aged youth will more easily grasp complex activities than intermediate grade children), and frustration tolerance.

- *How are participants relating to one another (group dynamics)?* In choosing and leading an activity for your group, of particular salience is how well group members are relating to one another. Some activities call for greater cohesion and cooperation (or can lead to greater frustration). Is your group ready for the level of challenge presented by a particular activity and/or would you like to push group members to a possible point of frustration (e.g., because they have enough process that you'd like to see if they can do some good conflict resolution)?

- *What is the energy level of the group?* Just like their counselors and therapists, clients ebb and flow with regard to energy. Does the group have enough energy for the anticipated activity? Do group members have too much energy for the activity (such that they are less likely to listen to instructions and stay with the task[s] involved)?

- *What areas and facilities do you have at your disposal? What equipment do you have?* Do you have adequate space for the activity or activities? Can you move outside or to a different space? Do you have some basic equipment or props on hand that might give you some flexibility? We typically have a small (or sometimes not so small) adventure activity bag with us. In it, we keep masking tape, soft balls or objects to toss, a tarp or tablecloth, and some other odds and ends. As you look to the 50 activities in chapter 7, you'll notice that with a few simple objects you have lots of options for different activities.

Formulating a Plan

As you answer the preceding types of questions, you can begin to formulate a plan as to the activity or activities that will best fit your group. As you continue with the planning process, remember the importance of overplanning to give yourself options, especially if you are planning a series of activities. By overplanning, you give yourself the flexibility to go in several different directions as the group or situation may dictate. We generally try to be prepared for three times as many activities as we are likely to have time for. This overplanning gives us lots of options and helps us relax so that, no matter what comes up, we'll have an idea of what to do next!

In addition to overplanning, we think it is critical to think about the sequencing of activities. You may recall from chapter 1 that sequencing, for us, means the order of activities either during a specific group or individual session or over the course of treatment. Regardless of the time frame, sequencing is a critical component for helping a group get the most out of an experience. As one counselor who uses adventure activities extensively put it, "We must remember that sequencing is the most important thing we do. Then we must remember that there is no sequence." In other words, leaders must have a general road map in mind that provides direction, but that is also flexible enough to allow for multiple paths to the same goal depending on the kinds of variables we've identified by asking the purpose-related questions.

Once you have identified your sequence of activities, we suggest you write it out. We're fond of using note cards—which can fit easily into your pocket. This written list of planned activities, as well as lots of other options, can serve as your overplanned script that details the order, options, potential timing, and other prompts to help you remember key points. You can also use this list to help you organize and prepare the equipment and space you will need to lead your activities. Sometimes we also use it to record our observations about the group in a specific activity.

I'm Ready, I'm Prepared—Here Come the Participants—Now What Do I Do?

As the participants in your group arrive, the practical things you need to focus on are assessing the group, learning names, and setting the ground rules of the experience and thus providing a context to the group.

Assessing the Group

Stay calm, take three deep breaths, and remember our standard answer: "It depends." Is this the first time you have seen or met the group? Is the group intact and functioning or are members new to one another? Will this be a recurring group or is this a one-time interaction? Will you have the group for an hour, 20 minutes, a full day? Will you see them again? How many times? What is the mood and energy level of the group? In the first few minutes that you meet a group, there are a number of different assessments you need to begin to make in order to make your time with the group worthwhile. We have found great value in assessing a group and then adjusting our choice of activities on the fly. This is one of the reasons we encourage you to overplan. Overplanning gives you preplanned options that let you be flexible in delivering the best interventions to facilitate your objectives.

The need for making a quick assessment of the group may mean having a quick activity for the group as soon as you start your time together. A quick Icebreaker (see chapter 1) can serve as a means to engage the group immediately, as well as a means to assess the group for the type of activities you have planned during your time together. For new groups, after an initial activity you might want to take a step back to learn names, talk about group rules, and provide a context for the group. For recurring groups, perhaps there is an activity the group members know you play at the start of every session, thus serving as a tradition or routine to help them make a transition to your time together.

Learning Names

It may seem obvious, but one of the most important components to successfully leading adventure activities is building an emotionally safe environment. This is a continuous process that we think begins with knowing other participants' names. Having everyone in the group learn names (including yourself) is a critical first step to making everyone feel welcome and a part of something. Use name games (e.g., I Can Do This!!, p. 113), name tags, or other creative means to assure that names are learned early in the process. We have found that "Hey you!" and "That guy over there" are not phrases that facilitate positive processing sessions. It really helps to know names.

Setting the Ground Rules of the Experience

We're guessing you have some experience in setting ground rules in groups. Establishing norms, etc., is not an atypical step in traditional counseling and therapy groups. That experience generalizes nicely to the process in groups in which you are using adventure activities. However, we also think there are a couple of fairly unique concepts that are of particular help in groups in which you use adventure interventions. One of these is the idea of a Full Value Contract.

Schoel and Maizell (2002) noted that the Full Value Contract is designed to ask the group "(1) to understand and/or create safe and respectful behavioral norms under which it will operate; (2) for a commitment to those norms by everyone in the group, and (3) to accept a shared responsibility for the maintenance of those norms" (p. 61). We often think of these as the typical classroom rules that primary grade school children develop for how they will be together in the classroom, or the kinds of values and mission statement that corporate groups develop to set the trajectory for the kind of culture they would like in their company. The Full Value Contract creates a context for sharing, learning, and being together. It helps group members identify what they are going to pay attention to while they are together. It creates the context for community. Schoel and Maizell also noted that a Full Value Contract should be developed in words that are understandable to all group members and should reflect "the unique spirit and purpose of the group" (p. 61). Although the basic principles of developing group ground rules remain constant, the means of developing the rules may be different, and establishing group ground rules can occur in a variety of ways.

Some leaders like to devote a lot of attention to this task the first time they meet with a group while others like to develop the group's rules incrementally. Specific techniques that can be used for creating group ground rules include

- *Hopes, Expectations, Concerns.* Have the group divide into three subgroups. Give each subgroup a piece of paper. One group will get a sheet that says "Hopes," another subgroup will get a sheet that says "Expectations," and the third will get a sheet that says "Concerns." Have the subgroups brainstorm their hopes, expectations, or concerns about the group (depending on their sheet). After a few minutes, rotate the sheets of paper to another subgroup. As subgroups get a new sheet of paper, have them review what has already been written and then add their own hopes, expectations, or concerns (depending on the sheet). After an additional few minutes, rotate the sheets again so every subgroup has had a chance to review and write on each sheet. Review the sheets as one big group making sure everyone understands what has been written.

- *Protect the Jewels* (p. 148). We sometimes use this activity to illustrate how the more people in the group are guarding the good stuff about the group, the easier it is to keep the good stuff going!
- *Community Puzzle* (p. 62). In this activity, the pieces of the puzzle can be important parts of the group's ground rules.
- *Develop a Formal Contract*. Have the group answer such questions as
    What are your expectations of yourself?
    What are your expectations of your fellow classmates?
    What are your expectations of your leaders?
- *Design a Totem Pole*. The pole signifies the rules and expectations of the group. This activity was written up by Henton (1996) as a kinesthetic, spatial, and artistic means for participants to define a group's guidelines and rules. It is most likely for use by longer term groups. First the participants determine the particulars of their group rules. Then participants identify the specific ways that they will value self, each other, and the experience. Next they design a totem that symbolizes their group. The group can use a written blueprint as the contract with each other, or the group can actually construct the totem out of wood, papier mâché, boxes, Styrofoam, or other recycled materials. After they have built the totem, participants can add words or pictures on each section to specify the behavior they are committing to for the experience.
- *Five Finger Contract*. For younger children, this activity is more directive, but it can be a good symbol for what the group is trying to work on. For each finger, have the group brainstorm what behaviors would fit with each concept. Once you have completed your discussions, you can have all participants give you a high five signifying their commitment to the ground rules. For groups meeting over multiple sessions, giving a high five is a quick way to review ground rules each time the group meets. In this scenario, each finger represents an important part of the contract:
    Pinky = Safety—it's the smallest and most vulnerable finger
    Ring finger = Commitment—willingness to let things go and not hold grudges
    Middle finger = Awareness of put downs
    Pointer finger = Taking responsibility instead of pointing blame
    Thumb = Agreement to work toward group goals
- *Definitions*. Create definitions for each of the following: play hard, play safe, play fair, have fun.

Challenge by Choice (Henton, 1996) represents another important concept in establishing group ground rules. Challenge by Choice for us includes the idea that how participants choose to challenge themselves in activities (or even in choosing not to participate in activities) is the choice of the participant. Not unlike any other client participation in the counseling or therapy process, Challenge by Choice highlights that participation is voluntary. However, unlike some other traditional counseling settings, adventure activities sometimes feel risky or challenging (e.g., having to get off the ground to get over the rope in Electric Fence, p. 67). Henton suggested that Challenge by Choice is based on these principles: (a) challenge or healthy risk taking promotes growth, (b) the individuals' basic needs for competence and accomplishment are positive motivation for learning, and (c) individuals possess the ability to determine their potential success in new situations.

We think that Challenge by Choice is one of the things that make adventure activities so powerful. Challenge by Choice places responsibility for participation, problem solving, assessment of risks, assessment of competence, and evaluation of what is worth doing and why with the client. We've found that when participants make choices they own their choices, in contrast to being told what they have to do. Challenge by Choice helps participants find their own strengths and limitations and take responsibility for their choices. The trick is to create an environment in which people feel comfortable to try new things if they want. One of the primary ways the leader does this is through sequencing. As we explained in chapter 1, we don't suggest that your first adventure activity with any group be a problem-solving initiative or trust exercise necessarily. We have found that if those activities are not sequenced up to (either through Icebreaker and Deinhibitizer activities or through other counseling interventions that develop cohesion, etc.), participants are less likely to participate. Because, for us, participation is never mandatory (but we'd obviously like participants to choose to participate), we try to emphasize sequencing in leading activities.

Enough With the Preliminaries. LET'S PLAY! Any Pointers?

Of course, that is what this chapter is all about! We want to encourage you to think about these areas as you begin your activity: getting ready to give instructions, giving instructions and assessing/adapting, monitoring safety, and transitioning to the next activity.

Getting Ready to Give Instructions

Clearly giving instructions is pivotal for getting an activity started quickly and in the right spirit. A first key to giving instructions successfully is to have multiple and various ways to engage the group, to get their attention, to get them ready to listen and focus. Some of our suggestions/techniques (based primarily on lots of mistakes we've made) are as follows.

1. *Position yourself* for giving directions as you prepare to give instructions. Make sure everyone can hear you, stay in front of the group (never place yourself in the middle of a group). Think about where participants are standing. For example, try not to have participants looking into the sun when giving directions.
2. *Use theme phrases* such as saying "Happy" and the group saying "Holidays"—if the session takes place in November or December. You can also have the group make up their own theme phrases.
3. *Consider calling for actions* by, for example, saying, "Clap once if you can hear me; clap twice if you can hear me; clap three times if you can hear me." As participants start to clap in unison the whole group quiets down and joins in the clapping. Other actions include raising your hand and having participants raise their hands and close their mouths in response. Or you can hold a handkerchief over your head and explain that as the handkerchief is free falling, the group members can make lots of noise, but once the handkerchief hits the ground they should be quiet and listening.
4. *Incorporate routines* for groups that meet multiple times. For example, start off sessions with the same activity every time, which can help the group ease back into their shared experiences. When the activity ends, the group knows it is time to focus their attention on you. Another example is using different types of whistles to bring the group to order. You can also have the group develop their own routines.
5. *Use your best stage whisper*, which will take participants a little off guard, we've found, and can help the group quiet down and get close together to begin to hear you.
6. *Use trigger words* to organize the group into a shape you'd like the group members to form (e.g., big circle, smaller circle, straight line) in anticipation of the activity. Make a game out of teaching group members these words, or make up your own. Remember to have some fun with this and perhaps even include the participants in making their own formations and trigger words. Our trigger words include
    a. *chicken noodles*. Group is to form a tight circle standing shoulder to shoulder—tightly touching, like noodles in a can of chicken soup.
    b. *chicken wings*. Group is to form a bigger circle by placing their hands on their hips and standing elbow to elbow with the person on each side.
    c. *flying chickens*. Group is to form an even bigger circle by stretching their arms straight out from their sides and touching the fingertips of the person on each side.
    d. *chicken and dumplings*. Individuals are to scatter, leaving each person room to swing his or her arms freely and not touch anyone else.

Giving Instructions and Assessing/Adapting

Once you are ready to give instructions, and the group is ready to hear the instructions, describe the rules or parameters of the activity as simply as possible. In some cases, you will want to give explicit directions, but in other cases you might want to be a bit vague to give the group more latitude in thinking through the challenge. Do take care to clarify explicitly any safety concerns (e.g., "Please stay away from the chairs, loose carpet, curbs") or specific rules that will help ensure a safe activity (e.g., "Please remember to move slowly at first because having your ankle tied to another participant's ankle can be pretty awkward"). In many situations, in addition to explaining the activity, it helps to also demonstrate the activity to help visual learners. In other cases, you may intentionally not want to demonstrate the activity as you won't want to hamper the group's creativity in figuring out how to do an activity on its own. If you do choose to demonstrate an activity, use participants to assist in the demonstration. You can also do practice rounds or play the first time in slow motion to make sure everyone understands the activity. If appropriate, you can include participants in deciding rule and procedural changes in general or for adaptations in playing the game or completing the activity.

When you have finished giving directions, get into the habit of asking if there are any questions. It may be clear for you, but make sure everyone is on the same page as you. In some cases, you may decide not to answer every question, especially if it relates to initiatives in which groups want to know the right answer but you want the group to figure it out together (or there is no right answer). If this is the case, tell the group that it is up to them, or clarify, or simply repeat the directions you already gave.

Once the directions have been given, get on with it and start the activity. However, you must still decide on what role you are going to play during the activity. Are you going to play? Observe? Observe from a distance? Give suggestions? There are definite advantages and disadvantages to each role, and it often depends on what you are trying to accomplish with the activity. For example, you might want to play to facilitate the action and involve everyone in the activity, or you might want to observe the activity to make either individual or group assessments. Whatever the case, be intentional about your role throughout the experience.

In addition to the leader's role during an activity, the leader must also monitor the group in terms of such things as energy, engagement, and group process. In response to these assessments, the leader can adapt the activity as the group dictates. Think about adapting activities as if you are at the controls of a stereo: you can change the base or treble, the balance of the speakers, the volume, etc. As a leader don't be afraid to fine-tune the experience for groups as well. Make the activity more difficult or easier to reengage, and help the group focus or keep everyone involved. For some more difficult challenges, it may be necessary to stop and come back to an activity at a later time when the group is better able to handle the challenge (e.g., when their energy level is not quite so frenetic). This type of *leading on the fly* is what makes leading adventure-based activities so challenging and fascinating: the leader is constantly being asked to assess the group and adapt to ever-changing situations. The leader must never be afraid to change the rules to fit the situation. For us, this concept of leading on the fly and being able to adapt activities is so important that we examine it in more detail in chapter 5.

Monitoring Safety

As we have already noted, safety is a critical part of leading groups. We have already tried to reinforce the importance of anticipating any safety concerns and giving and repeating explicit safety instructions. In addition, it is important for leaders to monitor safety throughout activities. With this in mind, we have found it extremely helpful to try and foster an environment that empowers everyone to monitor safety for everyone else throughout an experience. Sometimes, and especially with older groups, we describe three safety nets in an activity. The first safety net is you, the leader monitoring for safety. The second safety net is participants taking care of themselves. This is a natural extension of Challenge by Choice and taking care that all challenges are safe ones. The third safety net is participants monitoring one another throughout activities.

Techniques we've used to encourage and empower groups to monitor their own physical and emotional safety include the following:

- Before an activity begins, ask the group to identify potential hazards or unsafe conditions.
- When you as a leader see an unsafe condition, yell "FREEZE" or call a safety time out, so that the group freezes in place and evaluates safety. Ask the group, "What problems might exist and how might we address these problems?" Encourage everyone in the group to yell for a safety time out until the situation can be addressed.
- Use the Ripple Stop Technique. If anyone at anytime feels unsafe have him or her yell "STOP" as loudly as possible. Whenever anyone hears the word *stop*, he or she is to stop immediately and also yell "STOP" as loudly as possible, thus creating a ripple effect to stop the whole activity (Michaelis & O'Connell, 2000).
- Have the group evaluate the facilities or site for safety concerns before you even begin.
- Ask the group "What if" questions to have them begin to think about safety. Another good question set starts with "What do you think would happen if…?"

- Prior to beginning an activity, have everyone in the group raise his or her right hand and do a pledge to obey the rules and play safe!

Transitioning to the Next Activity

If you have more than one activity planned for a specific session, one of the challenges in leading is successfully transitioning to the next activity. After an activity is completed, and processed (if that is part of the plan), you are likely to need to consider several questions in your transition plan. These include, What is the energy level of the group? Do you need to re-energize the group and do a quick Icebreaker, or was the last activity high action and do you want to slow down the pace? What is the general mood of the group? Are they on a high from successfully completing an activity or feeling silly from a great Deinhibitizer? Have they just processed and are they really thoughtful and quiet? These types of questions help the leader identify what's next for this group. Once you have identified the activity you want to do next, you must think about how you will make the transition from one activity to the next.

Sometimes we use activities as specific filler or transition activities (e.g., Gotcha p. 79). These activities are often very different from whatever came immediately before and are almost a cleansing of the adventure palate. (Okay, that may be overboard, but you get our drift.) In some cases, you may be outside and have a distance to move for the next activity. In this case, you might think about such questions as, Does the group need a silent time to do some individual processing? or Is there a particular question or quote you want the group to discuss? For shorter distances and younger children, you might think about how you can keep the group together with everyone engaged. With these thoughts in mind, you might also think about how you can make the activity fun or challenging or engaging. Here are a few suggestions on how to move participants from one area to another in an orderly and fun manner:

- Sing a song as you go to a different activity.
- Walk silently.
- Pick a partner and walk.
- Follow the leader.
- Slow motion/fast forward.
- Have the group form an animal (e.g., elephant, bird) and then move together to the next activity.
- Have an ongoing story that you tell only during transitions.
- Use a large pretend television remote control and television to change the activity.
- Have participants take a Trust Walk (i.e., blindfolded walk being lead by other participants, p. 186).
- Have secret messages on a tape recorder (Mission Impossible style) regarding the next activity or announcements.

Closing Thoughts

It's hard to teach anything that can't be broken down into repeatable and unchanging elements. Driving a car, flying an airplane—you can reduce those things to a series of maneuvers that are always executed in the same way. But with something like leadership, just as with art, you reinvent the wheel every single time you apply the principle.
—Sydney Pollack (as cited by Bennis, 2003, pp. 125–126)

Becoming a dynamic adventure activity leader is an ongoing process. Don't be afraid to fail! Look at each experience as a tool for learning and improving the next time similar situations arise. Michaelis and O'Connell (2000) referred to this process as moving from unconscious incompetence to unconscious competence. Meaning, as we begin to lead we move from unconscious incompetence (not knowing what we don't know) to conscious incompetence (knowing what we don't know), to conscious competence (knowing what we know), and finally to unconscious competence (not knowing—or doing naturally what we know). Unconscious competence is when things flow for you as a leader, always making great decisions at the right time with seemingly little effort. Yet the best leaders don't stop at unconscious competence. They know they must continue to learn and look for ways to improve and develop skills that allow them to reinvent the wheel every single time they apply the principle. Here's to leading well and continuing to get better at it!

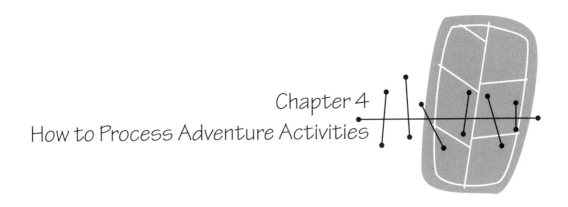

Chapter 4
How to Process Adventure Activities

This chapter explores the ideas for processing insights reached through participation in the activities and for helping participants generalize these insights into other relationships and situations. Before we talk about how to process activities, we should probably begin by asking WHY? Why process activities at all?

It may be a radical stance, but we say that you don't always process activities. We may be getting ahead of ourselves here though. What do we mean by *processing*? We typically mean talking about whatever game, activity, or adventure has just been completed. The typical scenario we might think of in processing an activity is to have a group (or subgroup) that has just played a game form a circle, so everyone can see and hear one another, and talk about the game they just played. Why do we process? We process because we are hoping that activity participants will come to some insight or awareness from the game or activity and that insight or awareness might be applicable beyond the game or activity, and might apply to other domains in life (e.g., school, family, or social situations). Through processing, we are hoping to facilitate the development of awareness and insight and promote the transfer of that awareness and insight to domains beyond the activity or game.

Now for our radical stance: we don't always process. Sometimes we think that it is unnecessary (maybe even counterproductive) to talk about the activity. We do typically process activities and think that you are likely to do so also. We do think it is usually helpful to process activities, and that's one of the main reasons we've included sample processing questions for all of the activities. However, we don't want to feel obligated to process (i.e., feeling as if the right way to do the activity includes obligatory processing) because sometimes we think it might be more facilitative not to.

One instance in which we think it might be better not to process is when the activity was primarily used as a bridge to another activity and/or an assessment activity (when we were setting a tone or checking to see what the group was like that day). For example, when we use an Icebreaker and have the time for another activity, we will sometimes not process the Icebreaker but process the next activity. Sometimes we will link activities together and process both activities after the second or third (if there were three linked together). In this way, we are processing all of the activities, just not in the typical way of talking after every activity. Another instance in which we might choose not to process an activity is when we perceive that the group or client really gets it. That is, when we have a sense that participants have come to awareness or insight and are likely to apply this to other domains, we will sometimes not process the activity. We think that this may be an effective way of staying out of the client's way. Although we think we're pretty good at this stuff (please don't burst our bubble), we're also aware that sometimes we get in our own way in trying to drive home a point and really get participants to make the connections. One other reason that we might hold back from processing a specific activity in which we think that the participants are making good connections is that we want to communicate respect. Part of what we mean here is that we think many participants can come to awareness and insight and apply that to their lives without our help. They are resourceful, and while we might be helpful at times, we (the facilitators/leaders/counselors) are not always absolutely necessary. Participants do the work.

With all that being said, we typically do process most activities. In the rest of the chapter we talk about some of the techniques we like to use and some of the things we consider in developing our processing strategies for different types of groups and activities. These include the size of the processing unit, what to focus on, and good processing techniques as well as using processing to help participants to think about their lives and the importance of metaphors.

What Is the Best Size for the Processing Unit?

One thing you are likely to get from us is that we do like to try and be creative and shake things up a bit. To that end, we like to process differently at different times with groups or clients. One of the ways we try to shake it up is to have different subunits process activities at different times. Obviously if you are doing activities with individual clients, any processing will be done by you and the client. However, in group situations, we use different processing units at different times. One of our goals in processing is to have group members talk to one another, not just to us. It is easy to get into the rhythm of asking a question and having the participants answer you. In this scenario (and we've been there), you look at the group and ask a question, and then the group looks at you while one person answers that question. This is typically not what we are looking for. In the nirvana of processing, we throw out a question and group members talk to each other about that question. This doesn't necessarily happen naturally, so we try to change processing subunits to facilitate it.

One natural subunit for processing is partners or pairs. The *paired share* is a great way to help participants begin to take part in processing. In this case, each participant simply finds a partner and responds to one or more questions from the leader/facilitator (e.g., the counselor asks the question and the pair of participants discuss their answers with each other). When we use the paired share, one goal is to make sure EVERYBODY is talking about the activity. Although the paired share doesn't necessarily accomplish the goal of everybody talking about the activity, it usually accomplishes the goal of everybody talking. The actual topic being discussed can sometimes vary (e.g., "When is lunch?" "I don't remember—hope it's better than yesterday's.") This raises an interesting question. What are you (the leader) doing while these pairs are processing? Although you could go for coffee, we've typically used this time to (a) plan the next activity, (b) clean up the last activity, and (c) eavesdrop on the pairs to see what they're talking about. We sometimes do (a) and (b) (plan and clean up), but nearly always do (c) (eavesdrop on conversations). And not only do we eavesdrop on these conversations, we're typically pretty obvious about it. Although this sometimes throws off pairs the first time we do it, in subsequent paired shares participants have gotten used to us leaning in and listening and do not seem to be deterred. Listening in also helps pairs stay on the topic because you are, in a matter of speaking, checking up on them. On occasion we may join a pair's conversation, though this is somewhat rarer. We have also found that, if we are eavesdropping in an obvious manner, it is good to at least cruise by and listen in at least briefly on every pair.

One of our goals for processing is to get everyone participating. This is a primary goal for the paired share also because we think that, once you've talked in one setting, you may be more likely to talk in another (e.g., the entire group processing an activity together); and that is what we are aiming for, all group members actively participating in the group processing of an activity. (It's a beautiful thing!) Another reason we sometimes use the paired share is to follow up a paired activity. If two participants have just done an activity as a pair, we sometimes like to have them talk about it just between the two of them. Further, we use the paired share sometimes as a kind of bridging activity to the next sequencing. For instance, we may have a group begin in paired shares, then have the pairs team up with another pair (making groups of four) to talk about another question. Sometimes we even have those groups of four double up to make groups of eight for another question. We recommend the paired share.

It makes sense that the next processing unit we talk about is the triad (three participants). We have found that, as facilitators, we can successfully ask triads to discuss somewhat deeper questions. In contrast to the paired share, in which the pressure is on one of the two people to always be speaking (or else have a potentially awkward silence), in triads there are just enough people to take the pressure off of each participant, but without having so many participants that one of them can successfully hide in the conversation.

Of course, one could reasonably build a rationale for almost any number of subgroups processing (e.g., half of the whole group for more intimacy than the entire group). Our encouragement to you is to be creative in who participants are talking to. As you mix up who is talking to whom about activities, you build group process and help participants get to know numerous other group members—and not simply those with whom they have a naturally affinity (e.g., girls talking just to girls). All of these variables will facilitate successful group processing, which is one of our main goals.

What Do You Focus On in Processing?

Now that you've decided what unit of processing you will be using in processing the activity, how do you do it? How do you facilitate participants' awareness and insight or, asked differently, what do you talk about? We know that you have more than adequate creativity and therapy mojo to ask great questions in processing. However, to spark some of that creativity and mojo we have included possible processing questions aimed at the activity's objective at the end of each activity's description. In this section, we'd just like to get you thinking about the kinds of things the facilitator can focus on in processing. The following list is adapted from Rohnke (1991).

- *Leadership and followership.* Did someone show leadership in the activity? If so, who? Why did they take the lead? How did you notice them doing it? How was this decided? How did you feel about it? Under what circumstances would this have happened differently? How would members like for leadership to be decided?
- *Support.* What is it? Where does it come from? In a group or family, how is support established? How does it shift from member to member? How is it communicated? How would members like the communication to change or improve?
- *Pressure.* Does it have a helpful or harmful effect? When? What determines whether it is helpful or harmful? How is it conveyed? How is it perceived? In a group or family, where does it originate? Are there patterns in how it develops?
- *Negativism–hostility.* How did the group or client express it? Why is it there? How does the counselor deal with it? In a group or family, what are the patterns that occur in who expresses it and who is the object of it? How do these relate to what happens in the daily life of participants?
- *Efficiency.* How can we achieve the step beyond "just doing it"? How will we know when it is "good enough"?
- *Competition.* Was there competition? Did it occur against self, against another team, against some nebulous other group or record of some kind? What is the client's comfort level with each of these? How can the counselor use it in a helpful way?
- *Fear.* What did the client fear? Were fears physical and/or psychological? How did the client deal with fears? How did the counselor and/or other members help/hinder? What did the client need to help with fears?
- *Joy and pleasure.* What was fun? Why? How could it have been more fun?

This is, for us, just a starting list, and you are likely to be able to think of lots of other great typical areas to process (e.g., competition, peer pressure). The processing questions we've included after activities follow in these types of themes with an aim toward insight and awareness around the objectives for the activity. You'll probably generate much better and more interesting questions, but we wanted to get your creativity sparked!

What Are Some Good Processing Techniques?

Processing techniques we use include props, scaling, limited descriptors, and experiential processing.

Using Props

Sometimes just for fun, or to shake things up, we use props to facilitate processing. What we mean by a prop is a physical object that might prompt the group to consider a specific question. For instance, on occasion after a problem-solving activity, we will whip a credit card out of our pocket (e.g., VISA, Master Card, preferably CANCELED) and ask, "Who would you like to give credit to?" Sure it is a little cheesy, but it gets the group thinking. (Who really would they like to give credit to for helping in the process, being encouraging, coming up with a good idea, staying positive, giving a helping hand, etc.?). We then pass the card around to whoever wants it, and each person who takes the credit card gives credit to another member of the group. This use of props usually gets a giggle or a groan, but does help us kick off some processing questions.

There are lots of props you can use. Some of our favorites include a ruler (How did the group Measure Up?—HA!), a cell phone (How was the group's Communication?), and a book of matches (Who gave the group a SPARK?). We like to use props as another way to engage groups and make the entire experience, the processing included, a fun time. We trust that you can think of lots of other props to use.

Using Scaling

Another technique we often use with participants is to ask for their rating or scaling on a variable related to the activity. In this technique, we typically ask participants to rate themselves or the group on a scale of 1 to 10 with 10 being "better" on whatever the variable is. For instance, we might ask the group to rate how successful the group was, how well they did at planning, how well they listened or communicated or worked together, or how much fun they had. (You can see that the list could go on forever.) We have found that the best questions relate to your particular reason for using the activity. Our typical strategy is to have each participant (often around the circle) give a number without any explanation. We usually let participants take a pass, but we do come back to them. We like to hear a number from everybody. Just for fun we will often, after we've heard all the numbers, throw out a comment, like "Okay, the average rating was 7.85—" which usually gets a look. (We've found that if we make up a number fairly close to what an average might be, some of the participants think that we actually did add the numbers up and figure the arithmetic mean in our heads—which we frankly think is hilarious).

Only after we have heard a rating from every person do we ask why participants gave it that particular rating. We are typically hoping that we can get a discussion started about the specific topic (e.g., communication, teamwork, planning, fun), and we have found that the ratings can give us a good start because each person has thought enough about the topic to assign the group or activity a rating. Another advantage of using scaling is that the entire group participates in the processing (which doesn't always happen). Granted, the only contribution a specific participant may make is to say a number (e.g., "8"), but that participant is still more actively involved in the processing than if he or she had not rated the activity. Participants have typically listened to the ratings of other participants, and each rating serves to inform the later discussion (even if a specific participant chooses not to elaborate on why he or she gave a particular rating). We have also found that speaking up once in a group (if only to say a number in response to a scaling question) increases the likelihood that the participant will speak up again later.

One of the things we're pretty careful not to do is punish the participant for speaking up. What we mean by that is that if a relatively quiet participant who is likely not to contribute to the discussion in response to an open-ended question does speak up and give a rating, we do not want to focus undue attention on the participant. It is easy to do this by asking a particular participant, "Why did you rate it an 8?" This may be attention the participant does not want, and the participant may learn that you get punished for speaking up at all. But if participants learn that they can speak up when they want to and only say as much as they want to, we think it creates more of the environment we'd like and increases the likelihood of increased processing participation later.

Limiting Descriptors

Another processing technique we often use, which is similar to the scaling just described, is to ask for a limited number of words. Typically we ask for descriptive words. For instance, we might ask participants to describe how they felt about the activity using three words or less. We find that giving participants a limit of descriptors (e.g., fun, challenging, and crazy) helps encourage participation in the processing. It also challenges each participant to think about the activity enough to describe it based on the prompt we gave. Again, as in scaling, we let participants pass, and we come back to them later. We haven't found anything magic about three words, and so sometimes we limit the descriptors to one word or two. We do encourage everyone to participate. One of the ways we do this is by not requiring three words (or however many we requested). We also happily let participants use the same words others have already used. (Sometimes an activity is just FRUSTRATING and that's the best word for it!)

One of the fun things about limiting descriptors is that sometimes those who are more reticent to participate in processing, but are willing to give one or two words, find it amusing that other participants who typically speak a great deal are initially a little frustrated by only getting three words (or less depending on your instruction). We also really like it when participants are almost bursting to tell you what was frustrating or fun or whatever descriptor they offered. We love active processing and so enjoy setting the group up to really talk about the activity in a productive way. We've found limiting descriptors in the initial processing a helpful technique to do this.

Experiential Processing

Another set of processing techniques we use regularly involves physical movement and expression to process. One example would be a simple "thumbs up, thumbs down, or thumb in the middle" to give an assessment of the activity (or some aspect of it). Again, we often like all of the participants to think about an aspect of the activity. We have found that if we ask people to show us how they feel about the group's communication, planning, teamwork, leadership, and process by giving us thumbs up, down, or in the middle, participants have to think a bit about how they're going to vote with their thumbs about the specific focus. It is also interesting for the group to see this snapshot of how others feel, through their thumb vote, about this specific focus. The thumb vote also helps us see how the group is perceiving the topic, and we can compare it to our perceptions (e.g., would we have voted thumbs up, down, or middle on the topic?). We like to follow up the thumb vote with a question such as, "What made it thumbs up (or down or middle) communication (or planning or whatever focus we initially asked about)?" This obviously invites all of the thumbs-up voters to chime in about their rationale for their votes. We do try and take care not to put a minority of voters on the spot to defend their votes. We have found that if a majority votes thumbs down, we can ask about the thumbs-down vote and usually get one or two thumbs-up voters to chime in about their perceptions. That makes it processing—which we love!

Another experiential processing technique we've sometimes used is to ask people to physically move in response to a question (with no explanation beyond their physical positioning). For instance, we might use an object on the floor (could be almost anything large enough to see) to represent the group and ask participants to move dependent upon how close they feel to the group. You can gauge participants' sense of the group cohesion by where they position themselves—pretty interesting for you and for the rest of the group to see. As in using other techniques, you can use lots of other prompting questions. Sometimes we will lay out a line on the floor (with tape or a rope or simply a line in the flooring) and use it as a continuum from weak to strong (or 1 to 10) and ask participants to physically position themselves on the line in response to some question. How much fun did we have today? How successful was the group? We identified listening as an area where the group could improve to be more successful: How was the listening in that activity? We've found that having participants move to begin their processing time helps them get into it a little more, shakes things up a little (which we often like), and is a little more fun (which we always like).

How Do I Use Processing to Help Participants Think About Their Lives (Not Just the Activities)?

As we said earlier, through processing we are hoping to facilitate the development of awareness and insight and promote the transfer of that awareness and insight to domains beyond the activity or game. This statement points toward our usual strategy in processing. First, we are hoping to facilitate the development of awareness and insight. We typically do that by focusing on what happened in the activity. As we've previously mentioned, we might use props, scaling, descriptive words, physical movement, and/or focused questions around a variety of themes. What we are hoping to do is help participants identify important issues, observations, and themes they noticed about themselves, others, or the group as a whole. We generally think of this as *personalization processing*. Schoel, Prouty, and Radcliffe (1988) described experiential learning as following the sequence of (a) experience, (b) reflection (what happened?), (c) generalization (now what?), and (d) application (so what?). We think of personalization, the initial phase of processing, as including reflection and some generalization. It is a focus on the experience and other potentially similar experiences. However, the key part of the processing is really application.

Clearly the point of processing adventure activities with children and youth is not so that they will get better at adventure activities (e.g., improve in their ability to communicate, problem solve, resolve conflicts, and appreciate others) so that they are even more successful in the next activity. The goal in processing adventure activities is to help children and teens apply insights from activities to other aspects of their lives at school, at home, and in social settings. We think this *application processing*, as we refer to it, is the key to helping participants transfer the learning from the activity to the world. It is a means of helping participants see how the fabricated adventure activities are related to real life. This application processing helps participants see the metaphorical value of activities.

Metaphors

One of the primary ways that we think about adventure activities is as metaphors. The reason that the activities lend themselves to developing insight and awareness that transfer to other life domains (beyond the activity) is that the activities are metaphorically connected with the rest of life. Remember that a metaphor is a comparison. A metaphor lays one thing beside another and says, "Look at how these things are alike!" Most of how we think and talk about our lives is metaphoric. Recently I (Jeff) was talking to Don and Terry, and I told them I was in a rut. Don quickly offered to get a towrope to pull me out, and Terry suggested that she would be willing to push! Actually, not so much—they didn't really think that I was in a literal rut and should be rescued (although nice of them to offer, eh?). They knew that I was speaking metaphorically about a pattern of behavior that seemed limited and difficult to get out of (like a car in ruts in the road). Because we tend to speak and think metaphorically about most of the aspects of our lives, using metaphorical activities can facilitate conversations about these aspects.

Some of the games and activities in this book have been played at camps for years. Often in those settings, facilitators will tell a story about a sea of peanut butter or nuclear waste that must be disposed of or some other fun story meant to engage the participants. Although we have nothing against peanut butter (though we do have issues with nuclear waste), we suggest that if you're going to tell a story, go ahead and tell a metaphorical story. For instance, in the activity Protect the Jewels (p. 148) we often talk about what the good stuff is that is being protected and the kinds of things that might ruin the good stuff. (Don't know what we're talking about? Go ahead and look ahead to see how the game is played! Really, we'll wait for you.) In this way, we front-load the activity with a metaphor. We basically tell participants before the game is played that the game actually represents the family or school or whatever we've set the metaphorical game to represent. We make the metaphor explicit, and then we talk about the activity afterward using that metaphorical language (e.g., "What was it like when two parents were protecting the good stuff?").

Another way that we use metaphors is to introduce the metaphor in the processing portion after the activity is over. In this way we back-load the activity with a metaphor. For instance, we might say that Helium Stick (p. 93) is like working together in a group and talk about similarities between those two things (e.g., what it was like to try and lower the tent pole and how hard it is to really work together in a group).

Finally, another way we use metaphor is to let the participants generate the comparison. Several authors (even us! see Kottman & Ashby, 2002) have argued that children and teens are natural metaphorical thinkers. We have found that children and teens can naturally and often brilliantly make metaphorical connections between activities and the rest of their lives. Because they are natural metaphorical thinkers, we find that with a little prompting (like front-loading or back-loading a couple of activities), participants will begin to make natural metaphorical connections. This metaphorical connection makes it easy to process activities because our natural goal in processing is to help participants transfer insights and awareness from the activity to other aspects of their lives.

Conclusion

We hope in this chapter you've gotten the flavor of processing. As we've said, there are sample personalization-processing and application-processing questions included for each activity in chapter 7. We think that if you try some of those questions and throw in some metaphors, scaling, paired shares, etc., you'll find a style and rhythm of effective processing that is all your own. We have found that after therapists and counselors make a few early connections, their counseling skills and creativity coalesce in ways that really facilitate clients' growth. With the simple ideas from this chapter, along with the sample processing questions, we think you're on your way!

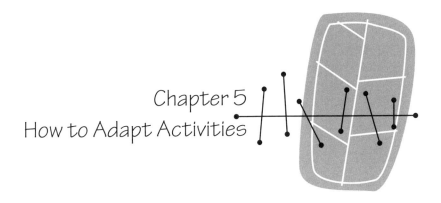

Chapter 5
How to Adapt Activities

As one of our favorite adventure leaders likes to say (with a smile), "When I am leading adventure activities for groups, they enter MY world." The phrase may strike you as a little odd, but we think it holds some truth. As the leader in adventure activities, you choose the activities for the objective you want to accomplish; you set the parameters for the activity (or purposely involve participants in this process) as well as change those parameters at any point during the activity (if it will help meet the objective). You are in ultimate control of the activity, and it is your world.

One of the ways that leaders do really make it their world is by adapting or tailoring activities for their specific group or objective. Just because you have a good activity (like those included in this book), please don't assume that it can't be made better. We have found it easy to learn an activity one way and then fall prey to the notion that it has to be played only in the form you learned it for it to work again (Rohnke & Butler, 1995). Although this may be occasionally true, it often isn't. There are so many variables that go into a successful activity that leaders must be prepared to adapt on the fly in response to the multitude of variables that play into the success of an activity both for the leader and the group. The purpose of this chapter is to prepare you to be ready to adapt an activity during the planning process as well as in the midst of the activity itself.

But Wait, I Thought the Activities in This Book Were Good Just the Way They Are: Why Might I Want to Change Them?

It is true we have tried to include activities that are ready to go as written (and the way we generally use them), but there are many reasons why you might want to change them either before you start or even during the activity. Some of these reasons include a need or needs to

- balance the challenge inherent in the activity with the abilities of the group;
- include participants with varying abilities (e.g., participant with a physical disability);
- incorporate different equipment because you don't have the specific equipment called for in the set up of the game;
- manage for environmental factors for an activity (e.g., weather, space);
- assure the safety of the group (both physical and psychological);
- include more or fewer players than the directions call for;
- address the dynamics of the group during the course of the activity;
- focus on a specific or different objective for the activity than listed;
- keep an activity novel and fun to play; and
- involve participants in the creative process of adapting an activity.

Okay, So I Might Have to Adapt Some Activities: Where Do I Start?

For us, it all begins with the question of Why? Why are you thinking about using a particular activity in the first place? When we know why we are doing something, we can figure out the how. For us, this means two things. First, as we plan the activities we want to use with our groups, we need to ask what we are trying to accomplish. How is the activity you have chosen going to help you accomplish this purpose? How can the activity be adapted in the planning process to better meet the objective or purpose you are trying to accomplish? Second, once the activity has begun, we want to monitor the activity to watch for opportunities to adapt the activity as it progresses to better meet the objectives for which the activity was chosen.

A Word of Caution

Before we go any further, we want to offer one word of caution about adapting adventure activities. Remember to be as intentional in the adaptation process as you are in all other aspects of leading adventure activities. Always be willing to adapt an activity to help you better meet the objectives you are trying to accomplish, but don't change an activity just because a group is struggling. The members of a group may find a particular activity is causing them to work harder than you or they expected. There is a difference between struggling to overcome the challenge in the activity and feeling unhappy with the activity itself. Rohnke and Butler (1995) reminded us that

> if a group is having to work hard and are disagreeing, not communicating effectively, arguing, etc. that may not be fun for them. However, it is part of the adventure experience…be careful to notice the difference between a group attempting to work through its problems and a game that, because it is inappropriate for a group, creates problems that do not need to be there. (p. 52)

If a group is struggling, that may give you really great things to process afterward or even in the middle! Remember that, for us, it is not really about the activity so much as it is about what we might get out of the activity that can be applied to the rest of life (see chapter 4).

Sounds Complicated. Do I Have to Be a Creative Person to Adapt Activities?

We have a long answer, but the short answer is NO. In our long answer, we refer you back to chapter 3, in which we talk about how to lead adventure activities. As a part of that discussion, we note that leading games and activities can be seen as part art and part science. The art of leadership includes the intangible qualities of leadership that are critical to success such as using sound judgment, integrating one's personality into activity leadership, and having a positive and upbeat attitude. These leadership elements are difficult to teach and are acquired and internalized over time. The science aspect of activity leadership can be taught and learned. It involves certain steps and much planning. When we think of adapting activities, we see this process as something that can be learned and developed. With your background and training, some initial experience leading activities, and some tips we will pass along in this chapter, you should be well on your way.

Our goal here is to suggest a number of different ways that you as a leader can adapt an activity to better fit your purpose. In each of these areas, we present a number of different questions that you can use to consider how you might change an activity. We think these questions will begin to help you feel comfortable with experimenting with activities and becoming comfortable inviting participants into YOUR WORLD as you introduce, lead, process, and maybe even adapt activities.

What Components of an Activity Can I Change?

As a general rule, any part of an activity is fair game to change or adapt. Morris and Stiehl (1989) identified a number of specific areas that you can work to change. These include players, objects (equipment), and organizational patterns. Let's explore each of these areas, examining the possibilities that each area offers to change a specific activity.

Players

As a leader planning an activity sequence, it is important to know a bit about the people who will be participating. In some situations you will have prior knowledge of group members; in other situations you will not. If you know very little about your group, you may use some Icebreakers to assess your group and get a sense of how the group interacts. Who are the leaders? Who are the followers? Does the group listen to you? To each other? How verbal is the group? What is their energy level? How about their impulse control? How do participants relate to each other? From this assessment (and from other good questions you will think of), you can begin to form a plan of how you might adapt an activity or activities to accomplish a specific objective.

Likewise, during an activity, you might adapt the activity to address or facilitate the dynamics of the group. Using adaptations can change the dynamics of the group or change the role that certain participants are playing in the group as well as change how the group is able to accomplish a certain task.

One adaptation we use regularly is assigning challenges or disabilities. In this adaptation the leader assigns specific challenges or tasks to participants that take away one or more of their senses or abilities. Challenges we use include

- blindfolding—when a chosen participant (or participants) loses his or her sight by being blindfolded during the activity. We have found that this often brings up issues of support, powerlessness, control, trust in others, and a sense of the unknown.
- muting—when a chosen participant is silenced and cannot speak during the activity. When we use this challenge, we often are able to process issues of communication, leadership, control, and reliance on others.
- paralysis—when a participant loses the ability to use a limb or limbs (often simulated by gently tying a hand to the side or legs together). This challenge often leads to discussions of teamwork, dependency, strengths and weaknesses, and empathy.
- connection—when participants are physically linked to each other. We will often tie participants' ankles together (like a three-legged race) or mandate that participants have to physically touch each other throughout the activity. It is easy to see how issues of cooperation, communication, consequences of behavior, and empathy are likely to come up in processing activities where you use connection as a challenge.

Remember, in assigning disabilities (as in all other aspects of the activity), it is your world. You can assign disabilities randomly; you can let the group or individuals choose; or you can strategically assign them. In assigning disabilities, you can obviously make it easier or harder for any one participant to be involved in an activity (e.g., muting a participant who is highly verbal). Although it is not necessarily our goal to intentionally frustrate a group (though it is a nice perk in some groups), assigning disabilities can make activities more challenging and take participants out of their normal roles. As long as this is strategic on your part, we say go for it! You may, though, need to be prepared for, as they say in the business world, some pushback.

Objects (Equipment)

Changing the equipment used in an activity can alter the activity a great deal. It can impact how players relate to each other, the overall challenge level of the activity, or even the objective of the activity (Rohnke & Butler, 1995). Equipment can be an attraction to play. Something novel and unusual arouses curiosity as well as a desire to participate. Likewise, the same old equipment can be a demotivator for people. For example, if someone brings out a basketball for a basketball game, there are a number of expectations that go along with this piece of equipment (e.g., this activity is only for tall people and better yet, coordinated tall people). One of our goals is often to use equipment that is unfamiliar to participants. When we use equipment that is unfamiliar (e.g., a rubber chicken in Flip Me the Bird, p. 76, or an old bike tire inner tube in Pass the Tire, p. 139) or when we use equipment in a different way (e.g., an old tent pole as a Helium Stick, p. 93), we think participants have fewer expectations and, as a result, may be more open to trying new activities.

Questions to think about in changing or adapting equipment include

- What objects are used in the game or activity? How can we use equipment in unique ways? As we have already stated, equipment can be an invitation to participate, and we need to think about what (if any) equipment we want to use in the activities we lead.
- How is equipment to be used in relationship to other equipment and participants? Sometimes we get in the mindset that all equipment has to be the same for everyone, but when we adapt activities we may want to use different equipment for different individuals (depending on their ability level). For example, if you are playing a game of Upchuck (p. 192), you may give some individuals bigger or smaller sized balls to make it easier or more difficult depending on their

ability. Another example using the game of Moon Ball (p. 130) relates to how equipment is used in relationship to participants. In Moon Ball, the intent is for the group to see how many times (hits) the group can keep a beach ball in the air. This could give taller people an advantage, and they might easily dominate the action as people are gathered around the ball. Yet a simple rule change (related to equipment and its relationship to participants), such as all players must touch the ball before a point is scored, can completely change the game.

- Can equipment be taken away, added, or modified from the activity? Absolutely! (And we like the way you think!) Consider again the Moon Ball activity (p. 130). If we added another beach ball (or two or three) and designated one ball as the one that we were using in counting the hits, while telling the group all balls must stay in the air, the game would be changed a great deal.

Organization Patterns

This section includes a number of different aspects related to the rules of the activity itself such as boundaries, how people move during the activity, and the organization of the activity. Questions to think about in changing or adapting the organizational structure of the activity include

- What types of movements are necessary? Can the movements in the activity be changed? For example, in Keypunch (p. 117), instead of having everyone walk, would it work to have everyone crab walk in an attempt to make the activity more difficult?
- What sequence do movements follow? Can you add or take away movement from the activity? How quickly or slowly do you want players to move? For example, in the activity Pairs Tag (on page 125 in our previous book, *Adventures in Guidance* [Kottman, Ashby, & DeGraaf, 2001]) we adapted this activity in several different ways. Initially the game involved everyone finding a partner, with one player in each pair designated It and thus having to avoid being tagged by her or his specific partner. Once tagged, the partners switch roles. We found we liked this game a great deal, but wanted to also play it indoors in a relatively small space. As a result, we had to slow down the action for safety purposes. So we adapted the activity by having everyone walk heel/toe. We also instituted the rule that if either partner runs into, or is run into by, someone else in the room, the person must stop and shake hands with that person saying, "I am terribly sorry. It will never happen again." By changing the way players moved and adding extra movement, we were able to slow the game down enough to safely play it indoors with a variety of players. In this case, we also think we made the activity more fun!
- What are the rules of the activity? How can they be changed? Rules are often associated with many of the elements already discussed in this section. They can relate to how players interact with each other or with equipment as well as what they are allowed to do in completing an activity. For example, in the activity Electric Fence (p. 67), rules may relate to the number of times the group can touch the rope (if at all), or how the last person has to get over the rope. Rules can change as time constraints change. If you are running out of time, you can change the rules in order to make the task easier so the group can complete the activity in the time allotted. Remember, it's your world.
- What are the physical aspects of the activity? What are the boundaries? How can they be changed? Changing the boundaries is a simple way of adjusting the activity level and the activity's difficulty or degree of challenge. For example, in the activity Heads or Tails (p. 90), the size of the playing area will greatly impact the time it takes to play the activity and the amount of energy the group uses. If the area is too big, it can produce fatigue, frustration, and a loss of camaraderie. If the area is too small, you can cramp the action, increase the risk of collisions, and limit the challenge level. But by finding the right playing area size, you create a much better chance for the activity to be successful and produce a desired outcome.

Lots of Good Questions to Stimulate My Thinking, But Do You Have a Process I Can Follow?

We are firm believers that you must find a process that works for you, so begin experimenting. We have said it before, but it bears repeating, always start by thinking about what you are trying to accomplish and work from there. With this in mind, here are some actions to take/considerations to help you in the development process.

1. Analyze the potential activity.
2. Identify what seems to work well or has a high potential for facilitating your goal.
3. Figure out what general changes are needed to accommodate your group, space, time, appropriate degree of difficulty/challenge, or objective.
4. Choose an adaptation that you think might facilitate the desired change (e.g., increasing or decreasing the degree of difficulty or challenge). We suggest that you don't try to do too much at once. Pick one adaptation, and try it to see if it works out. If you try to do too much at one time, it is hard to evaluate how each change impacted the group and the activity itself.
5. Keep notes on what works and what doesn't. (We often do this in the margin of the book next to the activity.) These notes can be extremely helpful as you return to an activity in the future.

Is Adapting an Activity Something Only the Leader Can Do? How About Involving Participants?

The answer to this question is, "It depends on what your objective is for a specific activity." If you want to encourage creativity and problem-solving abilities with the group, you may want to involve them in the process. Likewise, if you are trying to have a group be more inclusive, it may be helpful to have the group involved in the process of including everyone. In many ways, participants can be great partners in the adaptation process as they are participating in the activity. They can try multiple versions of the activity, evaluating as they proceed to come up with what seems to work well. In such an environment, it seems very appropriate to involve participants in the process.

When we involve participants in the adaptation of activities, we recognize the concept of cocreation inherent in our activities. The idea of cocreation relates to the shared meaning that emerges as leaders structure experiences, while at the same time stays open to the group as they cocreate the experience. This concept is exemplified when the leader structures the experience, but is also open to opportunities to help participants make the experience their own: It implies a dynamic balance in which the concepts are in constant motion yet remain in equilibrium. This is one of the variables that makes leadership such a dynamic process. It implies that leaders can correctly assess the group and decide how ready group members are to be involved in the process. There may be times when you as a leader simply make the changes you feel are necessary to meet specific objectives. At other times, you may involve the group (or even teach them) how to be involved in the adaptation process.

Okay, You Convinced Me, But I Tried to Adapt an Activity and It Didn't Work. Now What?

We feel your pain! We've been there, so we encourage you to keep trying, always remembering what you are trying to accomplish! If you find that adapting activities is not working for you, don't assume you don't have the gift or whatever it takes to alter a game. "Sometimes the insight for changing games is like a sixth sense. To develop the sense, you have to practice making changes. Practice and experience are required to do this well" (Rohnke & Butler, 1995, p. 57). This takes us back to the art aspect of leadership discussed in chapter 3. You must give yourself permission to experiment, to try new things and see if they work. This means being okay with failing (except in the area of safety) and trying again until you find what seems to work for you and your clients. We believe that as you become more comfortable with making changes, you will develop the intuition needed to adapt activities on the fly—and grow into the sense that it really is your world.

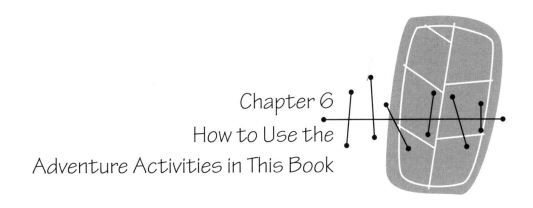

Chapter 6
How to Use the
Adventure Activities in This Book

Finally! In this chapter, we want to explain how to use the activities described in chapter 7. We want this book to be a resource for you to use with all sorts of clients in a variety of settings to accomplish specific purposes, and all while having FUN. To that end, we've organized the book in a specific way, and now we'd like to tell you how we organized the descriptions of the activities (on the off chance you haven't looked ahead to check them out already). We discuss in this chapter each component of the template used to organize each of the activities, how the activities relate to each guidance or treatment goal and objective, and how they can be cross-referenced and used to meet several different objectives at the same time. This seems a tall order, but we think we're up to it. (You'll obviously be the judge of whether we succeed.)

Name of the Activity

You'll note that every activity has a name. In response, you may be thinking, "Well, duh!" However, the name is a little tricky because activities, or variations of the activities, are often called by different names. For instance, what we call Keypunch (p. 117) we've also heard called Calculator. In some cases, we've tried to use the name we've heard most often (e.g., Keypunch), while in other cases we've just given the activity a name (e.g., Animal Crackers, p. 45) because we never heard the activity actually called anything. It is likely to have a name in some settings, but we're pretty fond of Animal Crackers. You may also note that we've tried to give credit when we have knowingly adapted an activity. Because our activity is an adaptation, we have typically given it a new name (but one close enough that you could find the original activity by name in the source we've identified).

Type of Activity

All of the activities in the book are divided into the categories of Icebreaker, Deinhibitizer, Trust, and Challenge/Initiative. As we highlighted in chapter 2, you might want to use these activities at different times for different purposes. To that end, we've included an appendix (Appendix C) that identifies the activities by type. By checking the grid (go ahead, we'll wait—), you can quickly identify activities that fall in to each category. Need a new trust activity? Check Appendix C.

Not to complicate things intentionally, but you may note that some of the activities have more than one type of activity (e.g., Icebreaker/Deinhibitizer) noted. These are not typos. Rather, it is our way of accommodating the fact that some of these activities do bridge categories. For instance, Cyclops Tag (p. 64) is identified as an Icebreaker/Deinhibitizer. This is because Cyclops Tag meets the criteria for Icebreaker (e.g., fun and emphasizing a success orientation), and it also pushes into the area of Deinhibitizers (e.g., extremely silly with some small personal risk). So when an activity seems to bridge categories, we simply list both in the description of the activity and place a "•" in the columns for both categories in Appendix C.

Grade Level

We have tried to set you up for success using the activities by estimating the earliest appropriate developmental age for each activity. We've done this by grade level because we have found that most of us think about children and teens in categories by grade (rather than age). Some of our grade levels estimates are field-tested. In some cases, we've tried the activities with younger children than we indicate is appropriate in this category, and it has not gone well. This may well have been our leadership, but we have attributed it, at least in part, to a mismatch of activity to developmental level of the client or group. With your talented leadership, you might try the activities with groups at a lower grade than is indicated in the description of a particular activity (e.g., Circles of Comfort, p. 59) with clients younger than third grade and be very successful. What we have tried to do is let you know what age groups have seemed appropriate for the activity in our experience. You may also note that we never give an upper age limit. This is, quite frankly, because we don't think there is one. We've done many of these activities with adults, and they often went swimmingly. We are guessing that you can imagine doing activities like Hug Tag (p. 102), Guidelines (p. 82), and Touch My Can (p. 178) with some adults you know. We also are guessing that you began to smile as you imagined them doing the activities.

Size of Group

In this category we try to help you estimate the optimal group size, or whether a group is needed, for the activity. Many of the activities work well with you and your individual client doing them. We've simply indicated that by giving "2" as the lower number of the range for the activity. For instance, you could easily do Chicks and Hens (p. 56), I Can Do This!! (p. 113), or Human Camera (p. 105) with your individual clients. In contrast, some activities are better suited to a group. We've tried to indicate the lowest number that still sets the group up for a successful experience. For instance, Helium Stick (p. 93) really goes best if there are at least 10 people.

We've also tried to give you an upper limit at which the activity seems to either be unmanageable or really loses its effectiveness. Some of the activities work pretty well no matter how large the group is (e.g., Gotcha, p. 79), but other activities have a clearer upper limit (e.g., Protect the Jewels, p. 148).

Activity Goals and Objectives

One of the exciting things about using adventure activities is that they can be framed, led, and processed to accomplish different purposes. In the activity descriptions in chapter 7, we identify the goals and objectives that might readily be addressed by the specific activity. The goals and objectives are based on the traditional goals that school counselors use in guidance programs and those used by mental health counselors in treatment programs. Appendix A provides a complete list of these goals and objectives.

Appendix B, Matrixes for Activity Goals, Objectives, and Grade Levels, then matches the specific goals and objectives to the 50 activities. One of the things we hope will make this book easy to use is that if you are interested in adventure activities and know that you want to help your client "develop skills for making and maintaining relationships," you can turn to Appendix B, see that, happily, that is the exact description for Goal 1G, and that there are 28 activities that can be framed, led, and processed to accomplish that objective. You may also notice that the activities have several, and in some cases a large number of, goals and objectives. We have found that you really can do the activity and accomplish different objectives based on how you frame, lead, and process the activities. Simply knowing what you want to accomplish at the outset helps you set up and lead the activity in a way to facilitate the objective. How you process the activity also makes a difference. We get to that part when we talk about the sample questions we include with each activity description.

Materials

In this section of the activity description, we identify all of the equipment or material you might need to do the activity. One of the fun things about these activities (and there are so many fun things, aren't there?) is that, for so many of them, no materials or equipment are needed (e.g., Mirror Mirror, p. 127; Stretching Story, p. 168). For most of the other activities, the materials needed are limited and readily accessible (e.g., masking tape for Guidelines, p. 82, and Traffic Jam, p. 182). Occasionally a specific piece of equipment really does enhance the game (e.g., rubber chicken for Flip Me the Bird, p. 76). When that is the case we've tried to indicate it. We love the portable nature of so many of these activities. It is particularly fun to do a session (from an hour to half a day) of these activities with absolutely no equipment. We can sequence from Icebreakers to Deinhibitizers to Trust activities to Challenge/Initiatives activities all without any equipment. Big fun!

Preparation

An important factor to consider when deciding whether or not to use an activity with a client or group is how much preparation is needed. Just as there is some variability in the ideal or appropriate number of participants for an activity, there is also some variability in how much preparation is needed before beginning the activity. Although many activities need no preparation (a beautiful thing), others require some thought and preparation. Often the preparation is to decide on, then mark, a boundary or distance to be crossed (e.g., Carry That Load, p. 52). The activities do not take significant preparation; if they did, this would, in our mind, defeat the purpose of using these activities intentionally as a part of your interventions with clients.

How to Play

Describing how to actually do the activities included in chapter 7 was, in some ways, our greatest challenge. What we've tried to do is give basic instructions that make it clear how the activity is done and how you might explain it to participants. One thing you may note is that we may have described the activity differently from how you have done it before. Obviously, feel free to do it your way! Or, if it sounds like fun, try our version.

Variations

As we've indicated elsewhere, there are lots of ways to do these activities. In this section of the activity descriptions, we've included some of our favorite variations. In some cases, the changes are small (e.g., try the activity in silence, no talking), but in other cases they are major (e.g., involving a significant rule change). Sometimes the variations can lend themselves to specific goals and objectives that might be accomplished with the activity. When that is the case we've indicated as much. We enthusiastically encourage you to shift rules and change the activities to best suit your client, group, objective, setting, or even mood.

Sample Personalization-Processing Questions

We include sample personalization-processing questions in the activity descriptions to stimulate your creativity around helping participants focus on their own experience in activities. The questions are designed to help participants think about how they experienced the activities and what they noticed about others in the group. As we said earlier, when we process, we are interested in facilitating the development of awareness and insight. Personalization-processing questions can help as they focus on what happened in the activity. These questions really address Schoel et al.'s (1988) idea of reflection (what happened?).

Please do note that these are just sample questions. We're pretty sure that you will come up with better ones for each activity with each client or group of clients. Giving the questions a specific contextual frame should make them have more of an impact. However, we wanted to get you thinking. Sometimes we have a sort of asker's block when it comes to processing questions. We hope that these sample questions will serve the purpose of inspiring you to generate even better questions.

It might be that some of these questions will be fine for use with your clients. You will obviously notice that some of the questions are geared toward specific goals and objectives. As a result, they may not work for your processing because you are planning to facilitate other goals and objectives.

As we said earlier, we don't always process activities. It may be that participants have gotten out of an activity what you had planned, and so little processing is necessary. If you do process, you will obviously want to gear the language to the appropriate developmental, cognitive, and verbal level of your participants. (This from one of us who used the word *ascertain* instead of *find out* with a kindergartener in a play therapy session—so it is a growing edge for some of us.)

Sample Application-Processing Questions

The purpose of sample application-processing questions is to stimulate your thinking about how to best help participants generalize their thinking and insights from the specific activities to other parts of their lives. As we said earlier, the point of adventure activities is to help participants apply insights and learning from these fabricated experiences to their lives. Application-processing questions really address Schoel et al.'s (1988) idea of generalization (now what?) and application (so what?).

As with the personalization-processing questions, the sample application-processing questions are a sample of what you might use to help participants generalize and apply learning. Because you will know the client or group and the specific context of the activity, you will probably generate specific application-processing questions. These questions are to spur your creativity and prime the pump of your own question generation.

Please do note that the sample questions are often relevant only to certain goals and objectives for the activity. As a result, if you do choose to use some of these questions, you will want to choose those designed to best facilitate the specific goals and objectives you had planned for the activity. You will also want to adjust the language of the questions to the developmental, cognitive, and verbal level of your participants as you are able to ascertain it.

Safety Concerns

The final category in the template describing activities is safety concerns. It is an obvious priority to be safe in all the activities. In this area, we highlight any general or specific safety concerns that might come up in the activity. Please note that any time there is movement (e.g., driving your car, walking down the street), there is inherent risk of people falling down, bumping into each other, twisting an ankle, or having some other accident. What we hope to do is help you anticipate any specific risk or safety concerns associated with the physical activity in the activity. We'd like to urge you to take these precautions seriously. In some cases, we have had close calls that have helped us outline safety concerns (one of the reason we don't have participants run in activities, although we used to). Also, when activities are safe (and you know they're safe), it is easier to have fun. Have fun!

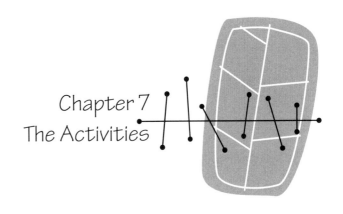

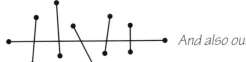

And also our favorite Marx Brothers movie!

Name of Activity: Animal Crackers

Type of Activity: *Deinhibitizer*

Grade Level: *Fourth grade and up*

Size of Group: *8 to 50*

Goal 1: Improve Communication and Relationship Skills

Objectives:

1B.   Express feelings clearly and constructively
1C.   Recognize and accept the feelings of others
1F.   Demonstrate willingness to trust others
1G.   Develop skills for making and maintaining relationships
1H.   Recognize and deal with peer pressure
1I.   Use communication skills to resolve conflict
1J.   Recognize the need for help and develop the ability to ask for it
1L.   Develop skills for effectively participating in groups

Goal 2: Increase Self-Awareness and Self-Acceptance

Objectives:

2A.   Explore personal attitudes and values
2C.   Develop ability to recognize negative self-talk
2D.   Develop skills in replacing negative self-talk with positive self-talk
2F.   Develop positive attitudes toward self

Goal 3: Develop and Apply Problem-Solving and Decision-Making Skills

Objectives:

3E.   Manage change and transitions in everyday life
3H.   Demonstrate effective coping skills for dealing with problems
3I.   Recognize when peer pressure is influencing decision making

Goal 5: Demonstrate Consistently Responsible Behavior

Objectives:

5D.   Develop coping skills for dealing with stress
5E.   Understand the need for self-discipline and self-control and how to exercise them

Goal 6: Enhance Positive Attitudes and Skills Related to Learning

Objectives:

    6A. Develop feeling of competence and confidence as a learner
    6B. Take pride in accomplishments
    6C. Accept mistakes as part of the learning process
    6E. Recognize that effort and persistence enhance learning

Materials: None

Preparation: None

How to Play:

1. Have the group stand and form a circle.
2. Explain that the object of the activity is to make an animal and that we'll do it in groups of three. Each of the three people will position themselves to make a part of an animal such that all three people together make the complete animal (e.g., two elephant ears on either side and an elephant trunk in the middle, three people making one elephant).
3. Explain, and model, what each animal part looks like. The animals we use are
    a. *the elephant.* To make the elephant, the person in the middle of the threesome brings his or her upper arm into contact with his or her nose (kind of an awkward position) so that he or she can wave the arm in front of the face to look like the trunk of an elephant. While the middle person is mimicking an elephant's trunk, the people on either side mimic the elephant's ears by bringing their arms up, one above the head and one about waist level (almost as if he or she was trying to show a half moon shape that pointed toward the people in the middle). There is your elephant. This is even more fun if the person in the middle makes elephant trumpeting noises while waving the trunk.
    b. *the giraffe.* To make the giraffe, the person in the middle of the threesome brings both hands up over the head and stands as tall as possible (we suggest tip toes). The persons on either side slide over so they are very close to the person in the middle and bend down with their hands on their knees. This looks like the tall neck of the giraffe and the legs on either side. There is your giraffe. We don't know any giraffe noises, but we would certainly award extra points (if points were included in this game) for them.
    c. *the frog.* Breaking out of the African motif, we include the frog. The frog is particularly fun. The person in the middle of the frog leans forward and sticks his or her tongue in and out (almost as if the frog was trying to catch flies). The people on either side of the frog's tongue do their best to imitate frog's legs. To do this each person leans in toward the person in the middle (those of us who are a little older often need to literally hold on) and raise the outside leg and kick it just a little. So, one frog's tongue going in and out and two frog's legs kicking.
4. Now after you have shown the various animal parts to participants, and everyone has practiced each part, explain the challenge. The challenge happens when one person—YOU to start with—is walking around inside the circle of participants. When you are ready, you point at one participant and say his or her name and then say one of the three animals (elephant, giraffe, or frog) and add "is my favorite animal at the zoo." For example, if you point at Maci and say, "Maci, elephant is my favorite animal at the zoo," it is then Maci's job to be the center of the elephant (the trunk, remember?), while the two people on either side of Maci need to become the elephant ears, thus forming the elephant, and all of this needs to happen before you finish saying "is my favorite animal at the zoo." Get the picture? The person in the middle is walking around inside the circle, the tension is growing, when suddenly the person turns, points at Juan and says, "Juan, frog is my favorite animal at the zoo!" As soon as the person says Juan's name, Juan knows he's going to have to be the center of one of the three animals (elephant, giraffe, or frog), and the people immediately to the left and right of Juan know that they're going to have to help form the animal, and that the three of them need to make the animal before the person inside the circle can finish saying "is my favorite animal in the zoo." If they don't finish in time, or if they get confused and do the wrong motion (and create a weird animal like an elephant with one ear and one frog leg), then the person who was pointed at, and whose name

was called (Juan in this example) gets to become the person inside the circle and that person takes Juan's place as part of the circle. So if Juan and the participants on either side get the animal right and do it before the person inside the circle can say "is my favorite animal at the zoo," then the person inside the circle stays inside the circle and continues calling names and pointing. However, if Juan, or either of the people beside him make a mistake or are too slow, then Juan comes inside the circle (even if he himself did the right thing quickly enough). This often makes for interesting things to process.

Variations:

There are other animals, but these are our favorites. We'd be interested to know yours!

Sample Personalization-Processing Questions:

1. How did you feel when the leader explained the activity? What did you anticipate would be the hardest part for you? What did you anticipate would be the easiest part for you? As you played the game, were your anticipations confirmed?
2. If you anticipated that you would be less than competent in this activity, how did that influence your behaviors? If you anticipated that this activity would be easy for you, how did that influence your behaviors?
3. Which was your favorite animal to make? What did you like about making that animal?
4. Which was your least favorite animal to make? What didn't you like about making that animal?
5. How important was working together in this activity? How did you increase the possibility that you would work together with the other two people in each triad?
6. How did you feel when you were one of the outside people in the triad and the person in the center of the triad didn't make his or her part of the animal correctly or didn't finish it in time and he or she had to go inside the circle? How did you express those feelings? What were some ways that could have expressed your feelings more clearly and constructively?
7. How did you feel when you were one of the outside people and you were the one who messed up, and the person in the center of the triad had to go inside the circle? How did you express those feelings? What were some ways that could have expressed your feelings more clearly and constructively?
8. How did you feel if you were the person in the center of the triad and one of your partners messed up, and you had go inside the circle? How did you express those feelings? What were some ways that you could have expressed your feelings more clearly and constructively?
9. What about this activity made it important to exercise self-discipline and self-control? How did that go for you?
10. On a 1 to 10 scale, what was your stress level during this activity? Did your stress level change depending on whether you were the center of the triad or one of the outside people? What did you find stressful in this activity? What made it stressful? What strategies did you use to cope with this stress?
11. Did you try to avoid being the person in the center of the triad? Why? How did you go about trying to avoid this? What was stressful about anticipating that you might be the person in the center of the triad?
12. How did peer pressure get played out in this activity?
13. Why did you have to trust the other people in your triad? What were some of the factors that influenced whether you trusted them?
14. How did you react to the silliness of this activity? Is silliness fun for you or not? What makes it fun (or not) for you?
15. How did you deal with it when you messed up? What did you learn from your mistakes? How did you apply what you learned from making a mistake the next time you were part of an animal?
16. How did effort and persistence pay off in this activity? Did mess ups inspire you to try harder or to give up? How could you use mess ups as a learning experience?
17. Did the members of your triad compare yourselves to the other triads? How helpful was making these comparisons?
18. How did it feel if you were in a triad that got an animal right?

19. How did the transition from animal to animal go for you? How did the transitions from animal part to animal part go for you? How did you handle those transitions? What did you learn during this activity about yourself and how you handle transitions?
20. Did you or anyone else in the group get angry during this activity? Did the anger result in any kind of conflict? How did you and/or the other members of the group deal with the conflict?
21. How was it for you to not be in control of the situation—to have to depend on others for success? How did you handle your reaction? How do you wish you had reacted?

Sample Application-Processing Questions:

1. Have you ever been in a situation when someone else might have to experience the consequences for your mistake(s)? What happened? How did you feel when that happened? What did you learn in this activity that you can use in situations like this in the future?
2. Have you ever been in a situation in which you were blamed for (or had to take the consequences) for someone else's mistake? What happened? How did you feel when that happened? What did you learn in this activity that you can use in situations like this in the future?
3. Some people master this task easily, and others do not. When you are in situations in which some people are mastering the task easily and others are not, how do you react? If you are one of the people who is mastering the task easily, what do you tell yourself about yourself and your abilities? If you are one of the people who is struggling with the task, what do you tell yourself about yourself and your abilities? What are some ways you could use positive self-talk to help yourself in these situations?
4. How do you usually handle transitions? How can you apply what you learned in this activity about your ability to make transitions in situations in which transitions are necessary?
5. What are some situations in which your anticipating something (usually negative) has a major influence on how you handle that situation? How can you apply what you learned in this activity about the impact of negatively anticipating something in these situations in the future? Positively anticipating something?
6. What situations or experiences in your life require working cooperatively with others? How can you apply what you learned in this activity to those other situations?
7. Which of the methods you used for managing stress in this activity would be helpful in other situations in your life? How can you use them?
8. Which of the methods you used for managing stress in this activity didn't particularly work? How can you avoid them in the future?
9. What are some other situations in which you might need to ask for help? How can you go about recognizing that you need help and asking for it?
10. How can you apply what you learned about dealing with mistakes in other situations in your life? Dealing with peer pressure? Feeling competent and confident as a learner?
11. What are some other situations in which, in order to be successful, you need to learn from past experiences? How can you apply what you learned in this activity to those other situations?
12. What are some other situations or relationships in which you compare yourself to others? When is comparing yourself to others helpful? When is it not helpful? What can you do to make it more helpful?
13. Are silliness and fun part of your value system? Why or why not?
14. In situations in which you feel angry or embarrassed, what usually happens? How do you deal with these situations? What did you learn from this activity that you can use in those situations?
15. How can you improve the way you handle situations in which you are not in control and must depend on others for success? What did you learn in this activity you can apply to those situations?

Safety Concerns: None

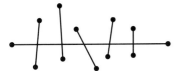

Do the Bump! No, not the 70s flashback bump, this Bump!

Name of Activity: Bump

Type of Activity: *Deinhibitizer; Challenge/Initiative*

Grade Level: *Third grade and up*

Size of Group: *8 to 16*

Goal 1: Improve Communication and Relationship Skills

Objectives:

1B. Express feelings clearly and constructively
1C. Recognize and accept the feelings of others
1D. Express ideas clearly and constructively
1H. Recognize and deal with peer pressure
1I. Use communication skills to resolve conflict
1J. Recognize the need for help and develop the ability to ask for it
1L. Develop skills for effectively participating in groups

Goal 3: Develop and Apply Problem-Solving and Decision-Making Skills

Objectives:

3A. Set personal goals
3B. Identify problems
3C. Demonstrate understanding of steps for solving problems and making decisions (gather information; explore alternatives and consequences; plan and take action)
3D. Evaluate decisions
3E. Manage change and transitions in everyday life
3H. Demonstrate effective coping skills for dealing with problems
3I. Recognize when peer pressure is influencing decision making
3J. Develop ability to identify alternative methods for solving problems and achieving goals

Goal 5: Demonstrate Consistently Responsible Behavior

Objectives:

5A. Acknowledge personal responsibilities
5D. Develop coping skills for dealing with stress
5E. Understand the need for self-discipline and self-control and how to exercise them
5G. Demonstrate respect for alternate perspectives

Goal 6: Enhance Positive Attitudes and Skills Related to Learning

Objectives:

6A. Develop feeling of competence and confidence as a learner
6B. Take pride in accomplishments
6C. Accept mistakes as part of the learning process
6E. Recognize that effort and persistence enhance learning
6F. Demonstrate dependability and initiative
6G. Develop the ability to share knowledge
6H. Develop critical-thinking skills

Materials: We usually use a knotted towel, but a very soft ball (even a beach ball) would also work. You need one towel (or ball) for each group of three.

Preparation: The only preparation is to mark the distance that the towel or ball must be tossed. (We usually mark off a distance of 10 to 15 feet).

How to Play:

1. This is a simple competitive game of catch with a couple of constraints.
2. Have participants get into groups of three.
3. Explain that one group member in each threesome should be the designated thrower while the other two members of the group are designated catchers.
4. Have the throwers stand 10 to 15 feet away from the two designated catchers.
5. Explain to the group that the designated thrower will loft the knotted towel or ball toward the catchers. The two catchers must catch the towel or ball without using their hands, arms, or shoulders. After catching the towel or ball they must transport it back to the thrower. After successfully catching the towel or ball (again, without using hands, arms, or shoulders) and delivering it to the thrower, the catchers take their places again 10 to15 feet away for additional throws and attempted catches.
6. If the catchers miss the towel or ball or break the rules by using hands, arms, or shoulders, they can simply pick up the towel and toss it back to the thrower.
7. Finally, let the teams know what the time limit is. We like to give a short initial time limit to see how many successful catches each team of three can pull off. After the first round, we often give teams a chance to brainstorm and process how to be more effective.
8. The winners, of course, get a big round of applause and the praise and admiration of their colleagues.[1]

Sample Personalization-Processing Questions:

1. How did it feel to not be able to use your hands, arms, or shoulders to catch the towel or ball? What did you do to express those feelings in a clear and constructive way?
2. How did you decide if your strategy for throwing and catching was effective? If it wasn't effective, how did your triad generate new strategies?
3. How important was working together in this activity? How did you increase the possibility that the three of you would work together?
4. How did you feel when you dropped the ball and had to start over? How did you feel when one of your partners dropped the ball and you had to start over? How did you express those feelings? What were some ways that could have expressed your feelings more clearly and constructively?
5. What were some ways that you recognized and accepted the feelings of others during this activity?
6. When there was conflict about a strategy for throwing and catching, how did you deal with the conflict? What were some ways you might have dealt with the conflict more effectively?
7. What did you do to contribute to the success of the group?
8. How did you decide whose ideas were used in planning your strategies?
9. How could you tell whether you needed help from the other people in your triad? What did you do when you needed help? How did you ask for help when you recognized you needed it?
10. What was your level of stress during this activity? If you had a time limit, how did this affect your stress level? What strategies did you use to cope with the stress involved in this activity?
11. What were your responsibilities to your partners in this activity? How did you decide what your responsibilities were?
12. Did you honor those responsibilities in playing this activity? If yes, what kinds of things did you do that you felt were responsible? How did you make sure your behavior was responsible? If no, what kinds of things did you do that you felt were not responsible? What kept you from being more responsible?
13. How did you deal with it if you thought you had made a mistake? What did you learn from your mistakes? How did you apply what you learned from making a mistake the next time you were throwing and catching?

---

[1] *Note.* Adapted from Rohnke, K. E., (1984). *Silver bullets.* Dubuque, IA: Kendall Hunt.

14. How did effort and persistence pay off in this activity? Dependability and initiative? Self-discipline and self-control?
15. In what ways did peer pressure affect the process? How did the members of your triad handle the peer pressure?
16. Did the members of your triad compare yourselves to the other triads? How helpful was making these comparisons?
17. How did it feel if your triad made many successful catches?
18. How did the transition from thrower to catcher go in your triad? How did you handle those transitions? Were there ways you could learn from your catching experiences the next time you were the person doing the throwing?
19. How did your triad handle conflicting alternative suggestions about how to make the catching/throwing process more successful?
20. How did the members of your triad decide how many successful tosses were "enough"?

Sample Application-Processing Questions:
1. What situations or experiences in your life require working cooperatively with others? How can you apply what you learned in this activity about cooperation to those other situations?
2. What are some situations or relationships in your life in which you feel handicapped in the same way you were in this experience by not being able to use hands, arms, or shoulders? How can you apply what you learned in this activity about working with handicaps to those other situations?
3. Which of the methods you used for managing stress in this activity would be helpful in other situations in your life? How can you use them?
4. What are some other situations in which you might need to ask for help? How can you go about recognizing that you need help and asking for it?
5. What are some other situations or relationships in which it might be important for you to be heard? How can you go about making sure that you are heard in those situations?
6. How can you apply some of the methods for communicating about feelings and ideas, encouraging cooperation, solving problems, and/or appropriately resolving conflicts that you learned/practiced in this activity in other situations?
7. How can you apply what you learned about dealing with mistakes in other situations in your life? Dealing with peer pressure? Dealing with stress?
8. What are some other situations in which, in order to be successful, you need to learn from past experiences? How can you apply what you learned in this activity to those other situations?
9. What are some other situations or relationships in which you compare yourself to others? When is comparing yourself to others helpful? When is it not helpful? What can you do to make it more helpful?

Safety Concerns: None except for the potential overenthusiasm of the catchers who could run into each other or other catchers.

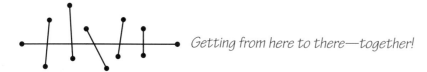

Getting from here to there—together!

Name of Activity: Carry That Load

Type of Activity: Trust; Challenge/Initiative

Grade Level: Fifth grade and up

Size of Group: 8 to 16

Goal 1: Improve Communication and Relationship Skills

Objectives:

1A. Demonstrate understanding of and apply basic communication skills (e.g., recognizing nonverbal cues, delivering "I" messages)
1B. Express feelings clearly and constructively
1C. Recognize and accept the feelings of others
1D. Express ideas clearly and constructively
1E. Listen actively to others
1F. Demonstrate willingness to trust others
1G. Develop skills for making and maintaining relationships
1H. Recognize and deal with peer pressure
1I. Use communication skills to resolve conflict
1J. Recognize the need for help and develop the ability to ask for it
1K. Recognize and verbalize needs and wishes
1L. Develop skills for effectively participating in groups

Goal 2: Increase Self-Awareness and Self-Acceptance

Objectives:

2C. Develop ability to recognize negative self-talk
2D. Develop skills in replacing negative self-talk with positive self-talk
2F. Develop positive attitudes toward self
2G. Recognize personal boundaries, rights, and privacy needs
2H. Identify personal and social roles

Goal 3: Develop and Apply Problem-Solving and Decision-Making Skills

Objectives:

3A. Set personal goals
3B. Identify problems
3C. Demonstrate understanding of steps for solving problems and making decisions (gather information; explore alternatives and consequences; plan and take action)
3D. Evaluate decisions
3F. Apply decision-making skills to resolve conflicts
3G. Apply decision-making skills in life situations
3H. Demonstrate effective coping skills for dealing with problems
3I. Recognize when peer pressure is influencing decision making
3J. Develop ability to identify alternative methods for solving problems and achieving goals

Goal 4: Increase Understanding and Valuing of Diversity

Objectives:

4A. Recognize and appreciate individual differences
4B. Develop an understanding and appreciation of own culture

4C. Demonstrate respect for others as both individuals and members of different cultural groups

4D. Acknowledge and appreciate similarities and differences across cultures and/or groups of people who have physical or learning differences

Goal 5: Demonstrate Consistently Responsible Behavior

Objectives:

5A. Acknowledge personal responsibilities
5B. Recognize whether behavior is appropriate and responsible
5C. Act in an appropriate and responsible manner
5D. Develop coping skills for dealing with stress
5E. Understand the need for self-discipline and self-control and how to exercise them
5F. Apply time management skills
5G. Demonstrate respect for alternate perspectives

Materials: None

Preparation: The only preparation is to mark the distance that the group must cross. It does not need to be far (e.g., across the room, 20 to 30 feet, or further).

How to Play:

1. This is an interesting challenge for groups. The directions are simple, but the problem feels complex.
2. The goal of the activity is for the group to move all its members across the room or open area (whatever distance you have marked or designated) as quickly as possible following these rules:
   a. To cross the open area, a person must be carried.
   b. The carrier must return and be carried him- or herself.
   c. The only person allowed to walk across the open area is the last person.
   d. If the carried person touches the ground while being transported, both those carrying and being carried must return to the start (or, as a variation, you can have the whole group start over).
   e. The number of people being carried and carrying can vary with the strength and/or imagination of the group (i.e., one to one is not the only way).
3. After you explain these rules to the participants, you may give them some time to plan before starting the clock.
4. Note that the better the planning, the faster the time for the whole group to get across. You can see how half of the group could simply carry the other half of the group piggy back and then the half of the group that acted as carriers could split in half with half of that group carrying the other half piggy back, etc., until the last person carries one other person across. There are also lots of other variations. Wonder which one is the fastest?[1]

Variations:

1. You can have the group try to beat their last time in a second or third try.
2. You can ask the group to set a time goal to accomplish the task.
3. You can challenge the group to move everyone in the fewest trips possible.
4. You can ask the group to set a goal of how few trips they can use to accomplish the task.

Sample Personalization-Processing Questions:

1. What was your reaction when you first heard the directions to this activity? How did you express your thoughts and feelings? Did your reaction change as the group discussed strategies? How?
2. What did you do to contribute to the success of the group? How did you feel about your contribution?
3. Did you feel heard as the group members worked on solving the problem? How did it feel when you were heard by other members of the group?

[1] *Note.* Adapted from Baack, S. (1989). *Adventure recreation.* Nashville, TN: Convention Press.

4. If you didn't feel heard, what was that like for you? If you had wanted to be heard by the other members of the group, what could you have done differently to make sure that you were heard?

5. Did you communicate your ideas and feelings effectively? If so, how did you go about doing this? If not, what prevented you from doing this?

6. What did you do in your role as a listener to make the process in this activity go more smoothly?

7. What role did trust play in this activity?

8. What process did the members of the group use to determine how to go about getting across the room? How did the group members decide whether a strategy was working? If a strategy wasn't working, how did the group members deal with that? How did you go about developing an alternative strategy when something wasn't working?

9. What were some of the ways that group members cooperated with one another to accomplish this task? How did cooperation help?

10. How did you decide whether to cooperate or not? How did your attitudes about cooperation influence what happened in the group? What about the attitudes of other group members?

11. How could you tell whether you needed help from other group members? What did you do when you needed help? How did you ask for help when you recognized you needed it?

12. What roles did various group members play in the process of getting across the room? How did the group members work out who was going to lead and who was going to follow? Did the roles change during the course of the activity? How?

13. How did you feel about being physically close and/or touching one another as you crossed the room? How much personal space do you need? How is this different from the other people in the group and their personal space requirements?

14. How did you feel about being carried? If you were one of the folks who carried others, how was this for you?

15. What was your level of stress during this activity? How did it change as time passed? If you had a time limit, how did this affect your stress level? What strategies did you use to cope with the stress involved in this activity?

16. When members of the group disagreed on strategies for crossing the room, how did you feel about the conflict? What did you do about your feelings? How did the group members resolve the conflict? What would have been some other ways to do this?

17. In what ways did peer pressure affect the process? How did the members of your group handle the peer pressure?

18. If you were feeling discouraged in this process, how did you deal with that? What did you tell yourself to motivate yourself to continue? If other group members were feeling discouraged, how did you interact with them about their discouragement?

19. How did you feel about it when the group made it across the room? How did you communicate those feelings to the rest of the group?

20. What were your responsibilities to the group in this activity? How did you decide what your responsibilities were?

21. Did you honor those responsibilities in playing this activity? If yes, what kinds of things did you do that you felt were responsible? How did you make sure your behavior was responsible? If no, what kinds of things did you do that you felt were not responsible? What kept you from being more responsible?

22. Were there times when you were telling yourself negative things about your ability to make a contribution to the group's success? What kinds of things were you telling yourself?

23. How could you have changed this negative self-talk to more positive self-talk? What kinds of positive things could you tell yourself?

24. If there was a time limit, how did you apply time management skills?

Sample Application-Processing Questions:

1. What are other situations or relationships in your life in which it feels as though you must carry others? What resources/strategies do you have to help you deal with these situations?

2. What are other situations or relationships in your life in which it feels as though you must be carried by others? What resources/strategies do you have to help you deal with these situations?

3. What are some other situations in your life in which you must have cooperation and help (work as a team) to be successful? How do you deal with these situations? How do you elicit cooperation and help?

4. How did the role(s) you played in this group resemble your role(s) in your family? In other groups? How do the other roles taken by various group members resemble roles taken by the other people in your life? What is your comfort level with these various roles?

5. How do you go about solving problems that are similar to the situation in this activity? Which of the methods for problem solving used by the members of your group would be useful in other situations in your life? How can you use them in these situations?

6. Which of the methods for managing stress that you or the members of your group used would be helpful in other situations in your life? How can you use them?

7. What are some other situations in which you might need to ask for help? How can you go about recognizing that you need help and asking for it?

8. What are some other situations or relationships in which it might be important for you to be heard? How can you go about making sure that you are heard in those situations?

9. How can you apply some of the methods for communicating about feelings and ideas, encouraging cooperation, solving problems, and/or appropriately resolving conflicts that you learned/practiced in this activity in other situations?

10. How can you apply what you learned about dealing with stress in other situations? Dealing with negative self-talk? Dealing with peer pressure?

11. What could you learn from this game that you could apply in situations in which it would be important to recognize and maintain your personal boundaries, rights, and privacy needs?

12. What are the rules (spoken or unspoken) about personal space and/or touching in your family? In your culture?

13. What are some other situations in which you have noticed differences in people's comfort levels about personal space and/or physical touch? What were the differences that you noticed? If someone else has different rules than you do about personal space, how can you handle this in an appropriate and respectful way?

14. What have you noticed about different cultural groups and their rules about personal space and/or physical touch?

15. What did you learn about your critical thinking skills that you can apply to other situations in your life?

16. What are some other situations in your life in which taking responsibility is important? How can you apply what you learned about taking responsibility in this activity to those other situations?

17. What are some other situations in your life in which trusting others is important? How can you apply what you learned about trusting others in this activity to those other situations?

Safety Concerns: If one person is carrying two others, ask spotters to walk with them. If the carrier weakens or stumbles, spotters may be needed.

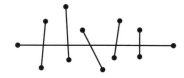

Okay—maybe feeding them sugar isn't such a good idea, but—
We like to play this game right after lunch to give them a little sugar
to combat those early afternoon doldrums.

Name of Activity: Chicks and Hens

Type of Activity: *Deinhibitizer; Trust*

Grade Level: *First grade and up*

Size of Group: *2 to 100 or more*

Goal 1: Improve Communication and Relationship Skills

Objectives:

   1E.   Listen actively to others
   1F.   Demonstrate willingness to trust others
   1G.   Develop skills for making and maintaining relationships
   1J.   Recognize the need for help and develop the ability to ask for it

Goal 2: Increase Self-Awareness and Self-Acceptance

Objectives:

   2C.   Develop ability to recognize negative self-talk
   2D.   Develop skills in replacing negative self-talk with positive self-talk
   2E.   Appreciate own uniqueness
   2F.   Develop positive attitudes toward self
   2H.   Identify personal and social roles

Goal 3: Develop and Apply Problem-Solving and Decision-Making Skills

Objectives:

   3H.   Demonstrate effective coping skills for dealing with problems
   3J.   Develop ability to identify alternative methods for solving problems and achieving goals

Goal 5: Demonstrate Consistently Responsible Behavior

Objectives:

   5C.   Act in an appropriate and responsible manner
   5D.   Develop coping skills for dealing with stress
   5E.   Understand the need for self-discipline and self-control and how to exercise them

Materials: Small candies, covered in a wrapper of some kind (like Kisses, Rollos, or Tootsie Rolls); blindfolds if you can't trust participants to keep their eyes closed

Preparation: Distribute the candy around the room in plain-sight locations.

How to Play:

1.   Divide the group into pairs; if there is an odd number of participants, you will have to play. (Oh, darn, that means you might have to eat some of the candy.)
2.   Have each pair determine which of them is older than the other. Whoever is the oldest becomes the "chick;" the youngest member of each pair is the "hen." (A little role reversal there.)
3.   Have the hens put the blindfolds on. (Or have them close their eyes if you think they are that trustworthy or if you don't have enough blindfolds.)
4.   Explain that there are pieces of candy secreted around the room and that their task is to find that candy (and eat it if they so desire—but not now—when everyone is done hunting). Further

explain that the hens are the only ones who can actually pick the candy up; the chicks are too young to be entrusted with the candy. But since the hens are blind, the chicks will have to help them find the candy and figure out how to pick the candy up and hold it until the end of the game when they can share it with the chicks.

5. Clarify that the only way the chicks can communicate with the hens is to make a noise that will let the hens know they are on the right track to get the candy. They cannot touch the hens to lead them to the candy (nor can they touch the candy), and they cannot talk to the hens using human language. After all, they aren't humans anymore.

6. Have each pair pick a distinct noise that is just for the two of them (you can clarify that it actually doesn't have to sound like a chicken, but it does have to be some kind of animal sound). They will want their noise to be unique so that the hens can figure out which chick is guiding them.

7. For younger children, you might want to mention that the closer their partner comes to the candy, the louder, faster, more frequently they might want to make the noise. Older kids usually figure this out for themselves, but if they are having trouble getting to the candy, you can add this suggestion later.

Variations:

With younger children, you can let the chicks touch the hens and guide them to the candy while they are making their noises.

Sample Personalization-Processing Questions:

1. How did you feel when you realized that this activity involved candy?
2. How did you feel when you realized that this activity required some people to be blind (or blindfolded)?
3. Which role did you find more appealing—chick or hen? What appealed to you about that role? What did you not like about the other role?
4. How did you feel about deciding which role you played based on who was the older person in your pair?
5. Why was listening important in this activity?
6. Hens: How do you think you did with listening? How could you have improved your listening skills?
7. How did your pair decide on the noise you were going to make? How did you make sure that your noise was unique?
8. Chicks: How did it feel to make that noise?
9. How did you decide whether your strategy for gathering the candy was successful? If you didn't think it was successful, what did you do to increase your effectiveness?
10. What role did trust play in this activity?
11. Hens: How did you ask for help when you needed it? How did it feel to ask for help? Chicks: How did it feel to be the one asked for help? The one providing the help?
12. What was your level of stress during this activity? How did it change as time passed? What strategies did you use to cope with the stress involved in this activity?
13. Did you ever compare your harvest of candy to that of other pairs? How did you feel when you compared yourself to others? Did you notice when others were comparing themselves to your pair? How did you feel about this?
14. If you were feeling discouraged in this process, how did you deal with that? If your partner or other pairs were feeling discouraged, how did you interact with them about their discouragement?
15. How did you feel about it when you successfully snagged a candy? How did you communicate those feelings to your partner?
16. What were your responsibilities in this activity? How did you decide what your responsibilities were?
17. Were there times when you were telling yourself negative things about your ability to successfully gather the candy? What kinds of things were you telling yourself?
18. How could you have changed this negative self-talk to more positive self-talk? What kinds of positive things could you tell yourself?
19. In what ways did you exercise self-discipline and self-control in this activity? Why was that important?

Sample Application-Processing Questions:

1. What are other situations or relationships in your life in which it feels as though you are wandering around blind, hoping for something positive to happen? What resources/strategies do you have to help you deal with these situations?

2. What are other situations or relationships in your life in which it feels as though you must be guided by others? How do you decide whether to trust others in those situations? What resources/strategies do you have to help you deal with these situations?

3. What are some other situations in your life in which you must have cooperation and help to be successful? How do you deal with these situations? How do you elicit cooperation and help?

4. How did the role you played in this activity resemble your role in your family? In other groups? What is your comfort level with this role?

5. How do you go about solving problems that are similar to the situation in this activity? Which of the methods for problem solving used by your pair would be useful in other situations in your life? How can you use them in these situations?

6. Which of the methods for managing stress that you used in this activity would be helpful in other situations in your life? How can you use them?

7. What are some other situations in which you might need to ask for help? How can you go about recognizing that you need help and asking for it?

8. What are some other situations or relationships in which it might be important for you to listen to others? How can you go about making sure that you are listening in those situations?

9. How can you apply what you learned about dealing with stress in other situations? Dealing with negative self-talk?

10. What are some other situations in your life in which taking responsibility is important? Trusting others? Comparing yourself to others? Exercising self-discipline and self-control? How can you apply what you learned in this activity to those other situations?

11. When are you the leader/guide (chicks) in your other relationships? How comfortable are you with that role? When are you the person who must be guided (hens) in your other relationships? How comfortable are you with that role? How do you decide which role to play? What is the downside for you in each of these roles? How can you get more comfortable with both of these roles?

Safety Concerns: The chicks need to be careful to keep the hens out of trouble—not leading them astray or letting them walk into walls, etc. Give them permission to touch the hens and guide them to safer territory if the hens are doing anything that might lead them into trouble.

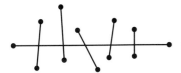 *Comfort for you, chaos for me! And vice versa—*

Name of Activity: Circles of Comfort

Type of Activity: *Icebreaker; Deinhibitizer*

Grade Level: *Third grade and up*

Size of Group: *1 to 100 and maybe more—if you have the room*

Goal 1: Improve Communication and Relationship Skills

Objectives:

1B.   Express feelings clearly and constructively
1C.   Recognize and accept the feelings of others
1D.   Express ideas clearly and constructively
1E.   Listen actively to others
1G.   Develop skills for making and maintaining relationships
1H.   Recognize and deal with peer pressure
1L.   Develop skills for effectively participating in groups

Goal 2: Increase Self-Awareness and Self-Acceptance

Objectives:

2A.   Explore personal attitudes and values
2C.   Develop ability to recognize negative self-talk
2D.   Develop skills in replacing negative self-talk with positive self-talk
2E.   Appreciate own uniqueness
2H.   Identify personal and social roles

Goal 4: Increase Understanding and Valuing of Diversity

Objectives:

4A.   Recognize and appreciate individual differences
4B.   Develop an understanding and appreciation of own culture
4C.   Demonstrate respect for others as both individuals and members of different cultural groups
4D.   Acknowledge and appreciate similarities and differences across cultures and/or groups of people who have physical or learning differences

Goal 5: Demonstrate Consistently Responsible Behavior

Objective:

5G.   Demonstrate respect for alternate perspectives

Materials: Open space to accommodate group and rope, webbing, string, yarn, tape, or some other marker to form to concentric (one inside the other) circle boundaries

Preparation: Use the marker (e.g., rope, string, tape) to form a larger circle and a smaller circle inside of it (sort of resembling a target). The outside circle should ideally be large enough that the entire group can stand shoulder to shoulder just outside of it.

How to Play:

1.   Explain to the group that the areas inside and outside the circles represent different degrees of comfort.

2. Tell participants that the area inside the smaller circle in the middle is the Comfort Zone. In this area, people are relaxed and perfectly comfortable. They are not anxious or stressed at all. We try to use developmentally appropriate language to describe comfort here (but some of us are used to only talking to other PhDs, which makes us very difficult to understand—even when we're not saying anything even remotely important).

3. Explain to participants that the area between the smaller circle and the larger circle is the Challenge Zone. In this area people feel challenged. They will generally experience a little more stress or anxiety than in the Comfort Zone, but it is not necessarily unpleasant, just uncomfortable.

4. Finally, explain to participants that the area outside the larger circle is the Chaos or Crazy Zone. In this area, people feel out of control and very stressed and anxious.

5. To review, inside the smaller circle is the Comfort Zone, where things are easy and comfortable. In the area between the inner circle and the outer, larger circle is the Challenge Zone, where things are a little stressful and somewhat uncomfortable. Outside the larger circle is the Chaos or Crazy Zone, where things feel out of control and unpleasant.

6. Now that you've explained what the different areas represent, have participants in the group move to a different area (i.e., Comfort, Challenge, or Chaos/Crazy) based on their reaction to a particular activity or experience.

7. The list obviously differs based on the kind, size, age, and experience level of the group. We've included things like speaking to a group of 100 other kids. Singing a solo. Taking a math pop-quiz. Attending a party where you don't know anyone. Flying on an airplane. Jumping out of an airplane. Asking someone on a date. Having the principal come on the loud speaker and tell the whole school that he or she would like to have you come to the office. Making a speech to your class. Having a new baby brother/sister. Moving to a new school. Meeting your boyfriend/girlfriend's parents. (This is only limited by your own imaginations—go wild!) (When we run out of ideas, after having done several, we ask the participants to generate ideas for the group to react to.)

8. Help participants think about whether the activity or experience would be "comfortable," "challenging," or "chaotic" for them and, based on their answers, have them move to that area of the circles.

9. Ask folks to notice who is in the same circle as they are—and who is not.

Sample Personalization-Processing Questions:

1. How did you feel about the different circles? Was there one circle you found yourself in most of the time? Which one? What do you think that was about? Which was the circle that felt most comfortable to you? (Hint: for lots of folks, that isn't actually the comfortable circle.)

2. Were there other activities or experiences you wish we had given you a chance to explore?

3. Were there patterns in the other people who reacted the same way you did (picked the same circle as you)? Were you with the same group of people every time or did it vary? What did you notice about people who tended to react the same way you did? What did you notice about the people who tended to react differently than you did?

4. What did you learn about yourself during this activity? Which of your reactions surprised you? What was surprising about them? Did you see any contradictions in your choices? How do you explain these contradictions?

5. What did you learn about the other members of your group? Did you see any contradictions in their choices? How do you explain these contradictions?

6. Did you notice any kind of peer pressure to go to a different circle than the circle you wanted to be in during this activity? If you felt peer pressure, how did you deal with it?

7. Did you want to talk about why you chose the circle you chose? If the group did talk about their choices, how did you feel about the way you expressed yourself?

8. Which was the activity or experience for which you had the most difficulty discerning where you wanted to stand? What was difficult about that one?

9. Which was the activity or experience for which you had the easiest time discerning where you wanted to stand? What made that one easy?

10. Was there anything in this activity that evoked negative self-talk? What was the negative self-talk about? How could you have replaced the negative self-talk with positive self-talk?

11. How did you feel when there was something that would have been chaotic for you and others reacted differently? How did you feel when there was something that would have been comfortable for you and others reacted differently? How did you demonstrate respect for alternate perspectives?
12. Did you notice any stereotypes you were holding about certain people in this process? How did your holding those stereotypes affect how you interacted with those people?
13. How did your family values and attitudes affect your choices in this activity? How did your cultural values and attitudes affect your choices in this activity?
14. Were there some activities or experiences that you felt would be chaotic for you that you would like to be more comfortable with? How can you get more comfortable with these activities or experiences?
15. If your group processed your choices, were you more of a talker or a listener? Is that the usual role you choose? What is comfortable about that role for you? What is uncomfortable about the other role?

Sample Application-Processing Questions:
1. In what other situations have you been surprised by others being uncomfortable or comfortable with something you didn't expect to evoke that reaction? What did that teach you about yourself? About your expectations of others?
2. How can you use what you learned about yourself in this activity to increase your levels of self-awareness and self-acceptance?
3. How can you use what you learned about your reactions to peer pressure to prevent yourself from being unduly influenced by others?
4. How can you use what you learned about your reactions to other people having different levels of comfort in certain situations to increase your respect for differences between people?
5. How can you work on improving your skill in the areas of expressing your feelings and listening to the feelings of others?
6. What are some ways you can learn to recognize and appreciate individual differences in situations in which people are not as overtly revealing as they were in this activity?
7. How can stereotypes affect your interpersonal relationships and attitudes toward others? What are some things you can do to prevent this from happening?
8. How can you learn to more fully appreciate your own uniqueness?

Safety Concerns: None

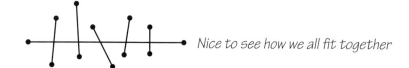

Nice to see how we all fit together

Name of Activity: Community Puzzle

Type of Activity: *Icebreaker*

Grade Level: *Fifth grade and up*

Size of Group: *8 to 24*

Goal 1: Improve Communication and Relationship Skills

Objectives:

1K.   Recognize and verbalize needs and wishes
1L.   Develop skills for effectively participating in groups

Goal 2: Increase Self-Awareness and Self-Acceptance

Objectives:

2B.   Identify and acknowledge personal positive traits, talents, and accomplishments
2E.   Appreciate own uniqueness
2F.   Develop positive attitudes toward self
2G.   Recognize personal boundaries, rights, and privacy needs
2H.   Identify personal and social roles

Goal 4: Increase Understanding and Valuing of Diversity

Objectives:

4A.   Recognize and appreciate individual differences
4C.   Demonstrate respect for others as both individuals and members of different cultural groups

Materials: Blank puzzle pieces, markers, and crayons

Preparation: You may buy ready-made puzzles from the following Web site (http://www.communitypuzzle.com), which offers two sizes: the community puzzle 48 pieces (24 border pieces and 24 four-inch-by-four-inch middle pieces) and the community puzzle junior (12 border pieces and 4 four-inch-by-four-inch middle pieces).
Or you can make puzzles by taking a large piece of poster board or even plywood and cutting a 1-inch border and then cutting puzzle pieces to fit within the border. If you create your own, you can cut the number of pieces you need for your specific group.

How to Play:

1.   The object of this activity is for each participant to decorate/label/identify a puzzle piece.
2.   We have found the ideal is when the puzzle has the same number of pieces as participants in the group. (Sometimes we've included ourselves. Sometimes we haven't.)
3.   We like to use this as a beginning activity so that the group can begin to see how they might fit together and how each person (piece) is important for a complete picture.
4.   We often instruct participants to draw on their piece of the puzzle
     a. something they bring to the group to make it successful, or
     b. something they need from the group to be successful.
     There are obviously many possible and varying instructions that you can give in order to get participants to depict what you'd like on their pieces of the puzzle. Run wild!
5.   After everyone has completed drawing on their puzzle piece, bring the group together and ask one person to place his or her puzzle piece on the ground and describe what he or she has drawn/depicted. Next, ask for someone whose puzzle piece interconnects with this first piece

to lay his or her piece down and describe it. Continue this process until all pieces are connected and described.

6. If the group has extra pieces (and/or if the puzzle has the border pieces available), we often ask the group to record group information on them. For instance, we've had groups write or depict group norms, expectations, and/or goals.

7. The completed puzzle can be used as a metaphor for the upcoming group experience and illustrates what every person brings to the group and/or what every person needs from the group to have a successful experience.

Variations:

It is also fun to reuse this activity again at the end of the experience. Each group member takes his or her piece of the puzzle from the original puzzle, and on the back side of each puzzle piece other members of the group write what they appreciated about this person throughout the experience. After everyone has had an opportunity to write down this information, it could be shared with everyone in the group.

Sample Personalization-Processing Questions:

1. How did it feel to acknowledge that you bring something that will help make the group successful?
2. How did it feel to tell the other members of the group what you needed from them to be successful?
3. Were you surprised at any of the things the other members of the group said? What surprised you? What was surprising about those things?
4. Were you surprised at any of the things you said about yourself? What surprised you? What was surprising about those things?
5. How was what you have to contribute unique? How was what you need from the group unique?
6. What role did you play in putting the puzzle together? How comfortable were you with that role?
7. What did you notice about the intersection of the puzzle pieces? Did these intersections have anything to do with interpersonal boundaries evident in the group?
8. What did you notice about similarities and differences among group members? How did the group members deal with these similarities and differences? What were some ways the members of the group could have been more respectful about differences within the group?
9. What did you learn about yourself from this activity?

Sample Application-Processing Questions:

1. In other groups in your life, how comfortable are you acknowledging that you bring something that will help make the group successful? How can you become more comfortable with this?
2. In other groups, how comfortable are you asking for what you need from the group? How can you become more comfortable with this?
3. In your relationships with your family, how comfortable are you acknowledging your strengths, talents, and accomplishments? In relationships at school? In relationships with friends? How can you become more comfortable with this?
4. What role(s) do you usually play in groups? Which of these roles are comfortable for you? What makes them comfortable? Which of these roles are uncomfortable for you? What makes them uncomfortable? How can you become more comfortable with roles in which you are currently uncomfortable?
5. What are some other groups in which noticing similarities and differences among group members is important? How do these groups deal with similarities and differences? What are some ways you and the other members of these groups could be more respectful about differences within the group?
6. What are your unique contributions to your family? To your class at school? To other groups? To the world?

Safety Concerns: None

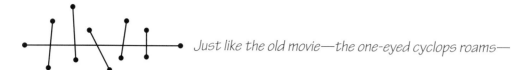 *Just like the old movie—the one-eyed cyclops roams—*

Name of Activity: Cyclops Tag

Type of Activity: *Icebreaker; Deinhibitizer*

Grade Level: *Third grade and up*

Size of Group: *2 to 100, maybe more—as long as it is an even number or, if not, if you're willing to play*

Goal 1: Improve Communication and Relationship Skills

Objectives:

1F. Demonstrate willingness to trust others
1G. Develop skills for making and maintaining relationships

Goal 2: Increase Self-Awareness and Self-Acceptance

Objective:

2H. Identify personal and social roles

Goal 5: Demonstrate Consistently Responsible Behavior

Objectives:

5A. Acknowledge personal responsibilities
5B. Recognize whether behavior is appropriate and responsible
5C. Act in an appropriate and responsible manner
5D. Develop coping skills for dealing with stress
5E. Understand the need for self-discipline and self-control and how to exercise them

Materials: Open space to accommodate the size of the group

Preparation: Marked boundaries if not easily apparent (e.g., inside the room)

How to Play:

1. Have each participant find a partner.
2. Explain that this is a game of tag that each person is playing only with his or her partner. One partner chases the other partner (walking, of course) and tags him or her. After the partner is tagged, he or she becomes It and chases the first partner. It is just a game of tag between the two partners.
3. So that the person who tags his or her partner has a chance to get away, after a person is tagged, that person must turn around two times and announce, "I'm It! I'm It! I'm It!" While the newly tagged person is turning around in circles, looking like a nut, the other partner should flee.
4. So far sounds like tag, right? "What about the cyclops part?" you ask. Well, to make the game more interesting, each person should close one eye. After one eye is closed, participants should place one of their hands in an O around their open eye (touching the tip of index finger of one hand to the thumb—try it). So, as I prepare to play, I may close my right eye, keep my left eye open, and place my hand around my left eye so that I can still see through that eye (but of course peripheral vision and depth perception is limited, presumably just like a cyclops).
5. The final instruction is to have participants raise their other hand (the one not surrounding an eye), palm out and elbow bent as a safety precaution.
6. Have the partner who will be It first begin by turning around two times and announcing, "I'm It! I'm It! I'm It!" And they're off!
7. Watch the chaos.

1. For younger or potentially more aggressive/clumsy groups, have them close one eye but keep both hands up for safety.
2. Again, for younger or potentially more aggressive/clumsy groups, or because it would be funny, have participants walk heel/toe (i.e., with each step you simply place the forward foot right in front of the other foot touching the heel of the forward foot to the toe of the other foot—little tiny steps). This slows progress down, is a little more awkward, and is often funny.

Sample Personalization-Processing Questions:

1. How did you feel about this activity? What did you like about it? What didn't you like about it? What was easy about it? What was difficult about it?
2. When you were the chasee, how did you feel when you got caught by the chaser? When you were the chaser, how did you feel when you caught the chasee? How did you feel during the transitions (changing from chasee to chaser and vice versa)?
3. Which role did you like best? What did you like about it? What did you dislike about the other role?
4. What were your responsibilities to your partner in this activity? What were your responsibilities to the group in this activity? How did you decide what your responsibilities were?
5. Did you honor those responsibilities in playing this activity? If yes, what kinds of things did you do that you felt were responsible? How did you make sure your behavior was responsible? If no, what kinds of things did you do that you felt were not responsible? What kept you from being responsible during this activity?
6. How could you tell whether other people perceived your behaviors as responsible? What kinds of feedback did you get from others (your partner, other people in the group, the leader) about whether you were being responsible during this activity? How did you react when you got this kind of feedback?
7. Did you feel that your partner was responsible during these activities? What kind of feedback did you give your partner about his or her being responsible (or not) during this activity?
8. How did your partner's ability to act in a responsible way affect your ability to trust him or her?
9. What about this activity made it important to exercise self-discipline and self-control?
10. What did you find stressful in this activity? What strategies did you use to cope with this stress?
11. What did you learn about yourself during this activity? What did you learn about your partner?

Sample Application-Processing Questions:

1. In relationships with friends, romantic partners (depending on the age, you probably don't want to include that part of the question with first and second graders, though times are a-changing), and family members, are you more comfortable as the pursuer or the pursued? What do you like about that role? How often do you play that role in relationships?
2. How often do you play the other role? What is uncomfortable for you about that role?
3. Are there other roles you play in your relationships (besides pursuer or pursued)? What are they? How often do you play these roles? How comfortable are you in each of these roles?
4. Have you observed other members of your family or your friends playing the role of pursuer or pursued? How do you feel about this when it happens?
5. What are some situations or relationships in which you feel that it is really important to act in a responsible manner? How do you handle these situations or relationships?
6. What are some times when you do not act as responsibly as you think you should? What do you think keeps you from being responsible in those situations? How could you handle those situations differently in the future?
7. How do you feel when you get feedback that you are not acting in a responsible manner? How do you react to this feedback? How is your reaction affected by who it is that is giving the feedback?
8. How do you handle situations in which friends or family members are not acting responsibly? What kinds of feedback do you usually give in these situations? How do you handle situations in which acquaintances or strangers are not acting responsibly? What kinds of feedback do you usually give in these situations?

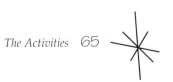

9. In what kinds of situations in your life do you feel the same kind of stress you felt during this activity? How can you apply what you learned about how you handle stress in this activity to those other situations?

10. What are some other situations in your life in which it is important to exercise self-control and self-discipline? How can you apply what you learned during this activity about your ability to exercise self-control and self-discipline to these situations?

11. What are some other situations in your life in which a person's willingness to act in a responsible manner can affect your ability to trust him or her?

Safety Concerns: Because peripheral vision and depth perception are limited, the chances of physical contact (bumping into one another) is increased. Reduced speed of locomotion (e.g., by requiring duck walking or heel/toe walking) may be helpful. DON'T let them play this game running.

Over the fence—without touching—all together!

Name of Activity: Electric Fence

Type of Activity: *Challenge/Initiative*

Grade Level: *Sixth grade and up*

Size of Group: *6 to 20*

Goal 1: Improve Communication and Relationship Skills

Objectives:

1A. Demonstrate understanding of and apply basic communication skills (e.g., recognizing nonverbal cues, delivering "I" messages)
1B. Express feelings clearly and constructively
1C. Recognize and accept the feelings of others
1D. Express ideas clearly and constructively
1E. Listen actively to others
1F. Demonstrate willingness to trust others
1G. Develop skills for making and maintaining relationships
1H. Recognize and deal with peer pressure
1I. Use communication skills to resolve conflict
1J. Recognize the need for help and develop the ability to ask for it
1K. Recognize and verbalize needs and wishes
1L. Develop skills for effectively participating in groups

Goal 2: Increase Self-Awareness and Self-Acceptance

Objectives:

2B. Identify and acknowledge personal positive traits, talents, and accomplishments
2C. Develop ability to recognize negative self-talk
2D. Develop skills in replacing negative self-talk with positive self-talk
2E. Appreciate own uniqueness
2F. Develop positive attitudes toward self
2G. Recognize personal boundaries, rights, and privacy needs
2H. Identify personal and social roles

Goal 3: Develop and Apply Problem-Solving and Decision-Making Skills

Objectives:

3A. Set personal goals
3B. Identify problems
3C. Demonstrate understanding of steps for solving problems and making decisions (gather information; explore alternatives and consequences; plan and take action)
3D. Evaluate decisions
3E. Manage change and transitions in everyday life
3F. Apply decision-making skills to resolve conflicts
3G. Apply decision-making skills in life situations
3H. Demonstrate effective coping skills for dealing with problems
3I. Recognize when peer pressure is influencing decision making
3J. Develop ability to identify alternative methods for solving problems and achieving goals

Goal 4: Increase Understanding and Valuing of Diversity

Objectives:

    4A.   Recognize and appreciate individual differences

    4B.   Develop an understanding and appreciation of own culture

    4C.   Demonstrate respect for others as both individuals and members of different cultural groups

    4D.   Acknowledge and appreciate similarities and differences across cultures and/or groups of people who have physical or learning differences

    4E.   Recognize how stereotypes can affect interpersonal relationships and attitudes toward others

Goal 5: Demonstrate Consistently Responsible Behavior

Objectives:

    5A.   Acknowledge personal responsibilities

    5B.   Recognize whether behavior is appropriate and responsible

    5C.   Act in an appropriate and responsible manner

    5D.   Develop coping skills for dealing with stress

    5E.   Understand the need for self-discipline and self-control and how to exercise them

    5G.   Demonstrate respect for alternate perspectives

Materials: Rope, string, webbing, yarn, or something else you can "string"

Preparation: You want to string the rope, string, webbing, or yarn at about hip-level of the average group member. This will be a boundary that the entire group must clear. You'd like it high enough that they cannot simply step over it. We often use the backs of chairs, park benches, trees, poles, etc., to tie the rope to. Note that the knots do not need to be strong or fancy. The participants are not supposed to touch the rope, so it should have no pressure on it at all.

How to Play:

1. This is a challenging activity in which the entire group must get over the rope without touching it.
2. To begin, have the entire group stand on one side of the rope.
3. We often use a metaphor and tell groups that they are stuck on that side of the rope and that the goal is to make their way to success on the other side of the rope. It is often fun to have them brainstorm about the kinds of things that typify success for them. We like to suggest that is what they are working toward, that those things are on the other side of the rope, and that if it were easy, everybody would be successful!
4. Explain that there are several rules for what is allowed as they try to travel from one side of the rope to the success side.
   a. All participants must go over the rope.
   b. No participant may touch the rope.
   c. No participant may touch whatever is supporting the rope (e.g., tree, chair, bench).
   d. Participants may not reach under the rope to help or assist.
   e. Participants must pass over the rope one at a time (for safety).
   f. Participants' heads must always be above their bums, bottoms, rears, behinds, butts (e.g., no diving or lifting participants where their heads are pointing down).
   g. No jumping of any kind is allowed. One foot must always be in contact with a surface (note that when there is a moment when neither foot is in contact with a surface, like the ground, you're jumping). We bend this rule a little at the very beginning as the first person is going over onto nothing. The point is that you can't jump, vault, or be thrown over. It must be a controlled and deliberate movement.
   h. You, the leader, can stop the group at any time for a safety reason (e.g., you are concerned about a lifting technique or that the person passing over the rope is going to have to jump which is, of course, against the rules).

5. If a participant breaks the rules, then that participant goes back over to the starting side. Sometimes we will say that, in addition, the last two people to come across to the success side must also go back to the starting side. Depending on how much time we have and the level of the group, we may say that if a rule is broken (e.g., someone touches the rope) the entire group must go back.

Variations:

1. This is a challenging activity, and we use several ending variations each time we do it. For instance, we may say that the last person coming to the success side can come under the rope or that for that last person the group can assist or support under the rope (but only for that last person). Our variations are usually an attempt to help a group be successful in the time frame allowed. We also do the activity regularly with no ending variation. It is challenging, but high functioning groups can readily accomplish the goals and achieve success.
2. Sometimes we give the group a time limit to accomplish the task.
3. We will sometimes lower the rope a little midway through the activity if it seems as if it is more challenging than we thought it was going to be. We particularly like to lower the rope a lot, then in just a minute or two raise it back up a little and to the actual height we wanted. This gives participants the idea that the height may change, in either direction. Success is hard to achieve and is sometimes a moving target.

Sample Personalization-Processing Questions:

1. How did your group define success? How did the group come up with this definition of success?
2. What parts of the group's definition of success corresponded to your personal definition of success? What parts of the group definition contradicted your own personal definition of success? How did you articulate this to the other group members?
3. What did you do to contribute to the success of the group? How did you feel about your contribution?
4. Did everyone feel heard as the group worked on solving the problem? How did it feel when you were heard by other members of the group? If you didn't feel heard, what was that like for you? If you had wanted to be heard by the other members of the group, what could you have done differently to make sure that you were heard?
5. Did you communicate your ideas and feelings effectively? If so, how did you go about doing this? If not, what prevented you from doing this?
6. What process did the members of the group use to determine how to go about getting over the electric fence? How did the group members decide whether a strategy was working? If a strategy wasn't working, how did the group members deal with that? How did you go about developing an alternative strategy when something wasn't working?
7. What were some of the ways that group members cooperated with one another to accomplish this task? How did cooperation help?
8. How did you decide whether to cooperate or not? How did your attitudes about cooperation influence what happened in the group? What about the attitudes of other group members?
9. How could you tell whether you needed help from other group members? What did you do when you needed help? How did you ask for help when you recognized you needed it?
10. What roles did various group members play in the process of getting over the fence? How did the group members work out who was going to lead and who was going to follow? Did the roles change during the course of the activity? How?
11. How did you feel about being physically close and/or touching one another as you crossed the fence? How much personal space do you need? How is this different from the other people in the group and their personal space requirements?
12. If you had to be lifted over the fence, how did you feel about this? If you were one of the folks who helped to lift others over the fence, how was this for you?
13. If you were one of the people who messed up and had to start over, how did you feel about this? What did you tell yourself about your competence when this happened? What did you tell yourself about other group members when this happened? What did you communicate to the rest of the group when mistakes happened?

14. If you were one of the people who had to come with the person who messed up and redo your crossing, how did you feel about having to do it again even though you had not messed up? How did you express your feelings to the group?

15. What was your level of stress during this activity? How did it change as time passed? If you had a time limit, how did this affect your stress level? If the leader changed the height of the rope, how did this affect your stress level? What strategies did you use to cope with the stress involved in this activity?

16. When members of the group disagreed on strategies for getting over the fence, how did you feel about the conflict? What did you do about your feelings? How did the group members resolve the conflict? What would have been some other ways to do this?

17. In what ways did peer pressure affect the process? How did the members of your group handle the peer pressure?

18. What personal positive traits and talents did you bring to this process, and how did you use them to help in getting everyone over the fence?

19. If you were feeling discouraged in this process, how did you deal with that? What did you tell yourself to motivate yourself to continue? If other group members were feeling discouraged, how did you interact with them about their discouragement?

20. How did you feel about it when the group made it over the fence? How did you communicate those feelings to the rest of the group?

21. What were your responsibilities to the group in this activity? How did you decide what your responsibilities were?

22. Did you honor those responsibilities in playing this activity? If yes, what kinds of things did you do that you felt were responsible? How did you make sure your behavior was responsible? If no, what kinds of things did you do that you felt were not responsible? What kept you from being more responsible?

23. What did you notice about differences in the various group members in the way they went about this task? What did you notice about similarities in the various group members in the way they went about this task?

24. Did you notice any stereotypes you were holding about certain people in this process? How did your holding those stereotypes affect how you interacted with those people?

25. If there were participants with physical challenges, how did the group deal with those?

Sample Application-Processing Questions:

1. How do you define success in other situations in your life? How can you apply what you learned in this activity about yourself and the way you think and feel about success to other situations in your life?

2. What are other situations or relationships in your life in which it feels as though you must cross an electric fence? What resources do you have to help you deal with these situations?

3. What are some other situations in your life in which you must have cooperation and help (work as a team) to be successful? How do you deal with these situations? How do you elicit cooperation and help?

4. How did the role(s) you played in this group resemble your role(s) in your family? In other groups? How do the other roles taken by various group members resemble roles taken by the other people in your life? What is your comfort level about these roles?

5. How do you go about solving problems that are similar to an electric fence that must be crossed? Which of the methods for problem solving used by the members of your group would be useful in other situations in your life? How can you use them in these situations?

6. Which of the methods for managing stress that you or the members of your group used could be helpful in other situations in your life? How can you use them?

7. What are some other situations in which you might need to ask for help? How can you go about recognizing that you need help and asking for it?

8. What are some other situations or relationships in which it might be important for you to be heard? How can you go about making sure that you are heard in those situations?

9. How can you apply some of the methods for communicating about feelings and ideas, encouraging cooperation, solving problems, and/or appropriately resolving conflicts that you learned/practiced in this activity in other situations?

10. How can you apply what you learned about dealing with mistakes in other situations? Dealing with negative self-talk? Encouraging persistence and flexibility? Dealing with peer pressure? Dealing with stress?

11. What could you learn from this game that you could apply in situations in which it would be important to recognize and maintain your personal boundaries, rights, and privacy needs?

12. What are the rules (spoken or unspoken) about personal space and/or touching in your family? In your culture?

13. What are some other situations in which you have noticed differences in people's comfort levels about personal space and/or physical touch? What were the differences that you noticed? If someone else has different rules than you do about personal space, how can you handle this in an appropriate and respectful way?

14. What have you noticed about different cultural groups and their rules about personal space and/or physical touch?

15. What did you learn about your critical thinking skills that you can apply to other situations in your life?

16. What are some other situations in your life in which you could notice and celebrate your own uniqueness? Your talents, abilities, contributions? Your successes?

17. What are some other situations in your life in which stereotypes might affect how you respond to other people? How can you apply what you learned in this activity to those situations?

Safety Concerns: The obvious concern is that people are off the ground as they come over the rope because it is too high to simply step over. As the leader, you have an important safety monitoring role in this activity. First, you need to vigorously enforce all the safety rules (e.g., no jumping, one person over at a time). Second, you need to spot any person who is in the air. You can take it as your job and/or assign others in the group to help spot also. Although the group is not technically supposed to use your help to get over, they are supposed to use your help to stay safe. Watch knees and ankles for those who come down hard. Make sure that if someone is being lifted that there is adequate support on both sides of the rope.

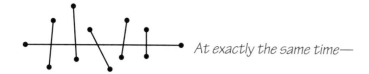 *At exactly the same time—*

Name of Activity: Everybody Up!

Type of Activity: *Trust; Challenge/Initiative*

Grade Level: *Second grade and up*

Size of Group: *2 to 200 (no kidding—works with 200), just need an even number*

Goal 1: Improve Communication and Relationship Skills

Objectives:

1A. Demonstrate understanding of and apply basic communication skills (e.g., recognizing nonverbal cues, delivering "I" messages)
1B. Express feelings clearly and constructively
1C. Recognize and accept the feelings of others
1D. Express ideas clearly and constructively
1E. Listen actively to others
1F. Demonstrate willingness to trust others
1G. Develop skills for making and maintaining relationships
1I. Use communication skills to resolve conflict
1J. Recognize the need for help and develop the ability to ask for it
1K. Recognize and verbalize needs and wishes
1L. Develop skills for effectively participating in groups

Goal 2: Increase Self-Awareness and Self-Acceptance

Objectives:

2C. Develop ability to recognize negative self-talk
2D. Develop skills in replacing negative self-talk with positive self-talk
2F. Develop positive attitudes toward self
2H. Identify personal and social roles

Goal 3: Develop and Apply Problem-Solving and Decision-Making Skills

Objectives:

3A. Set personal goals
3B. Identify problems
3C. Demonstrate understanding of steps for solving problems and making decisions (gather information; explore alternatives and consequences; plan and take action)
3J. Develop ability to identify alternative methods for solving problems and achieving goals

Goal 5: Demonstrate Consistently Responsible Behavior

Objectives:

5A. Acknowledge personal responsibilities
5B. Recognize whether behavior is appropriate and responsible
5C. Act in an appropriate and responsible manner
5E. Understand the need for self-discipline and self-control and how to exercise them

Goal 6: Enhance Positive Attitudes and Skills Related to Learning

Objectives:

6A. Develop feeling of competence and confidence as a learner
6B. Take pride in accomplishments
6C. Accept mistakes as part of the learning process
6E. Recognize that effort and persistence enhance learning
6F. Demonstrate dependability and initiative
6G. Develop the ability to share knowledge
6H. Develop critical-thinking skills

Materials: None

Preparation: None

How to Play:

1. The goal is for the pair to sit down, touch toes, hold hands, and stand up at exactly the same time.
2. Have participants pair up, face their partners, and sit down.
3. Have participants sit with their feet flat on the ground in front of them, touching the toes of their partners.
4. Have participants grasp their partners' hands.
5. Now, as they continue to hold hands and with their toes touching, tell them that their task is to stand up together. It is helpful to mention (as a small casual hint toward success) that the closer one's heels are to one's rear end (or bum for those of you in the UK) the easier it is to stand up. We often also mention that the key is to pull like crazy and work at standing up together rather than simply using the other person's weight to pull you up and forgetting to pull him or her up also. (This happens almost every time to somebody—hence the name EVERYBODY Up.)

Variations:

1. After pairs have successfully stood up, have the pairs join other pairs to make groups of four. Using the same rules—sit down, touch toes, hold hands, stand up at the same time—have the group of four take on the task. Note that partners can reach across the hands of the other pair to pull themselves and their partners up. (You can suggest this or let the group discover it.)
2. If groups of four have been successful, have participants form larger groups (e.g., 8, 16, 32, or any other number—go wild!). Just so you know—after about four participants, it is very hard to reach directly across to your partner over others' arms. Participants' arms are just not long enough. Wonder how they'll work it out?

Sample Personalization-Processing Questions:

1. What did you feel/think about your chances for success when the leader first explained the rules? How did you express your thoughts and feelings?
2. What did you do to contribute to your pair successfully standing up? How did you feel about your contribution?
3. If you and your partner didn't successfully stand up, how was that for you? How did you handle this failure? What did you tell yourself about yourself and your abilities related to this failure? What did you tell yourself about your partner related to this failure? How could you have dealt with this more constructively?
4. How important was communication between you and your partner in this activity?
5. Did you feel heard by your partner as you worked on standing up? How did it feel when you were heard by your partner?
6. If you didn't feel heard, what was that like for you? If you had wanted to be heard by your partner, what could you have done differently to make sure that you were heard?
7. Did you communicate your ideas and feelings effectively? Did you communicate your needs and wishes effectively? If so, how did you go about doing this? If not, what prevented you from doing this?

8. How did you do as a listener in this activity? How could you have improved your listening?
9. What role did trust play in this activity? What could you and/or your partner have done to enhance trust between the two of you?
10. What process did you and your partner use to determine how to go about standing up together? How did you and your partner decide whether a strategy was working? If a strategy wasn't working, how did you and your partner deal with that? How did you go about developing an alternative strategy when something wasn't working?
11. What were some of the ways that you and your partner cooperated with one another to accomplish this task? How did cooperation help?
12. How did you decide whether to cooperate or not? How did your attitudes about cooperation influence what happened between you and your partner?
13. How could you tell whether you needed more help from your partner? What did you do when you needed more help? How did you ask for more help when you recognized you needed it?
14. What roles did each of you play in the process of standing up together? Did one of you need to be the leader to have your pair be successful? If so, how did you work out who was going to lead and who was going to follow? Did the roles change during the course of the activity? How?
15. How did you feel about being physically close and/or touching one another as you worked to stand up together? How much personal space do you need?
16. If you and your partner disagreed on strategies for standing up, how did you feel about the conflict? What did you do about your feelings? How did you and your partner resolve the conflict? What would have been some other ways to do this?
17. If you were feeling discouraged in this process, how did you deal with that? What did you tell yourself to motivate yourself to continue? If your partner was feeling discouraged, how did you interact with him or her about the discouragement?
18. What did you learn from failed attempts to stand up? How did you use that learning to perfect your strategies for standing up?
19. How did you feel about it when you and your partner stood up? How did you communicate those feelings to your partner?
20. What were your responsibilities to your partner in this activity? How did you decide what your responsibilities were?
21. Did you honor those responsibilities in playing this activity? If yes, what kinds of things did you do that you felt were responsible? How did you make sure your behavior was responsible? If no, what kinds of things did you do that you felt were not responsible? What kept you from being more responsible?
22. Were there times when you were telling yourself negative things about your ability to stand up? What kinds of things were you telling yourself?
23. How could you have changed this negative self-talk to more positive self-talk? What kinds of positive things could you tell yourself?
24. What part did effort and persistence play in whether you and your partner were successful in standing up together?
25. How did you feel if the leader suggested doing this activity in bigger and bigger groups?
26. How did you apply what you had learned from standing up with your partner to the bigger groups? Were there times when applying what you had learned from the pairs exercise didn't work with the bigger group? How was that for you? How did you cope with that?
27. Did you and/or your partner look around and compare yourselves to others? How did that affect you and your efforts?

Sample Application-Processing Questions:

1. In what other situations or relationships in your life does it feels as though you must work with other people to make something happen? What resources/strategies do you have to help you deal with these situations?
2. What part does cooperation play in these situations or relationships? How do you elicit cooperation and help?
3. How did the role you had with your partner resemble your role in your family? With friends? How flexible are you about roles?

4. How do you go about solving problems that are similar to the situation in this activity? Which of the methods for problem solving used by you and your partner (or the members of the bigger group) would be useful in other situations in your life? How can you use them in these situations?

5. What are some other situations in which you might need to ask for help? How can you go about recognizing that you need help and asking for it?

6. What are some other situations or relationships in which it might be important for you to be heard? How can you go about making sure that you are heard in those situations?

7. What are some other situations or relationships in which it might be important for you to be a good listener? How can you go about making sure that you are using effective listening skills in those situations?

8. How can you apply some of the methods for communicating about feelings and ideas, encouraging cooperation, solving problems, and/or appropriately resolving conflicts that you learned/practiced in this activity in other situations?

9. How can you apply what you learned about dealing with negative self-talk?

10. What could you learn from this game that you could apply in situations in which it would be important to share information with others?

11. What did you learn about your critical-thinking skills that you can apply to other situations in your life?

12. What are some other situations in your life in which taking responsibility is important? How can you apply what you learned about taking responsibility in this activity to those other situations?

13. What are some other situations in your life in which trusting others is important? How can you apply what you learned about trusting others in this activity to those other situations?

14. How do you react when something you have learned can't be transferred to a similar situation? How can you learn to more effectively adapt to the new circumstances?

15. What are some other situations in which you have felt like a failure? How have you handled these situations? How can you apply what you learned in this activity to those situations?

16. What are some other situations or relationships in which you compare yourself to others? What has the impact of those comparisons been on you and/or your relationships? How can you apply what you learned in this activity about comparing yourself to others to those situations or relationships?

Safety Concerns: Enthusiastic participants can pull their partners over, and tumbles can occur.

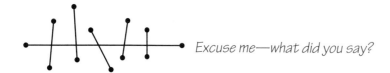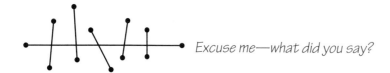
Excuse me—what did you say?

Name of Activity: Flip Me the Bird

Type of Activity: *Deinhibitizer*

Grade Level: *Fifth grade and up*

Size of Group: *6 to 30*

Goal 2: Increase Self-Awareness and Self-Acceptance

Objectives:

    2C.   Develop ability to recognize negative self-talk
    2D.   Develop skills in replacing negative self-talk with positive self-talk
    2E.   Appreciate own uniqueness
    2F.   Develop positive attitudes toward self
    2G.   Recognize personal boundaries, rights, and privacy needs
    2H.   Identify personal and social roles

Goal 5: Demonstrate Consistently Responsible Behavior

Objectives:

    5A.   Acknowledge personal responsibilities
    5B.   Recognize whether behavior is appropriate and responsible
    5C.   Act in an appropriate and responsible manner
    5D.   Develop coping skills for dealing with stress
    5E.   Understand the need for self-discipline and self-control and how to exercise them

Materials: You basically need a rubber chicken. That's right, you need a rubber chicken. They are actually readily available. Who knew? Party and novelty stores and Web sites have them. There really is no substitute in this game. In addition, they are great fun at parties and make outstanding gifts!

Preparation: Mark off an appropriate boundary for this game of tag.

How to Play:

1.   This is a simple game of tag—with a variation of Base in which participants are safe from being tagged as It.
2.   As always, this is, for us, a WALKING game.
3.   Explain to participants that it is a game of tag (a WALKING game of tag) and that you (the leader) will begin by being It. If you tag another participant, that participant becomes It and needs to chase (WALKING) other participants.
4.   The important addition to a normal tag game is that participants are safe from being tagged as It only if they are holding the rubber chicken (the bird).
5.   If participants are in danger of being tagged, they simply need to shout, "Flip me the bird!" as a sign that they'd like to have the rubber chicken tossed to them so they are safe from being tagged It.
6.   We recommend you (the leader) being It first. If you are It, you can move toward people and help them catch on to the value of shouting, "Flip me the bird!" to avoid being tagged.
7.   We also recommend a somewhat tight space so that participants often need to shout, "Flip me the bird!" to escape being tagged.
8.   As in other games of tag, we like to slow down the transition of the person who is newly tagged and to alert all the participants to who is It now. We often have the newly tagged person raise his or her hands and jump up and down while yelling, "I'm It! I'm It! I'm It!" It's also funny.

Variations:

We can't think of any. It's pretty funny just to hear people shouting, "Flip me the bird!" which we don't hear that much in other settings. Go figure.

Sample Personalization-Processing Questions:

1. How was this game of tag different for you than other games of tag?
2. How did you decide whether to ask someone to flip you the bird?
3. If someone asked you to flip them the bird, how did you decide whether to do it or not?
4. If several people wanted you to flip them the bird, how did you decide which one to flip the bird to?
5. Were there times when you were telling yourself negative things about your ability to tag others? Your ability to keep away from a person trying to tag you? What kinds of things were you telling yourself?
6. How could you have changed this negative self-talk to more positive self-talk? What kinds of positive things could you tell yourself about your abilities in this game?
7. How was it to have permission to say something (like, "Flip me the bird!") that would usually get you into trouble?
8. Which role did you like best: taggee or tagger? What did you like about it? What did you dislike about the other role?
9. What were your responsibilities to the group in this activity? How did you decide what your responsibilities were?
10. Did you honor those responsibilities in playing this activity? If yes, what kinds of things did you do that you felt were responsible? How did you make sure your behavior was responsible? If no, what kinds of things did you do that you felt were not responsible? What kept you from being more responsible during this activity?
11. How could you tell whether other people perceived your behaviors as responsible? What kinds of feedback did you get from others (other people in the group, the leader) about whether you were being responsible during this activity? How did you react when you got this kind of feedback?
12. What about this activity made it important to exercise self-discipline and self-control?
13. What did you find stressful in this activity? What strategies did you use to cope with this stress?
14. What did you learn about yourself during this activity?

Sample Application-Processing Questions:

1. In relationships with friends, romantic partners, and family members, do you like to have a clear distinction between the pursuer and the pursued? How do you deal with it when there isn't that clear distinction?
2. Which role do you like best, pursuer or pursued? What do you like about that role? How often do you play the other role? What is uncomfortable for you about that role?
3. Are there other roles you play in your relationships (besides pursuer or pursued)? What are they? How often do you play these roles? How comfortable are you in each of these roles?
4. How do you handle it when you are in situations or relationships in which the roles are not clearly defined?
5. What are some other situations or relationships in which you might be telling yourself negative things about yourself or your abilities? How do you feel in these situations or relationships?
6. What are some strategies you have used for shifting your self-talk in a more positive direction? How could you more consistently apply these strategies to situations in your life in which you tend toward negative self-talk?
7. What are some situations in your life in which you might have permission to do or say something that would normally get you into trouble? How do you feel about those situations? How do you handle those situations?
8. What are some situations or relationships in your life in which you feel that it is really important to act in a responsible manner? How do you handle these situations or relationships? How can you apply what you learned in this game to those situations?

9. What are some times when you do not act as responsibly as you think you should? What do you think keeps you from being more responsible in those situations? How could you handle those situations differently in the future?

10. How do you feel when you get feedback that you are not acting in a responsible manner? How do you react to this feedback? How is your reaction affected by who it is that is giving the feedback? By how the feedback is delivered?

11. How do you handle situations in which friends or family members are not acting responsibly? What kinds of feedback do you usually give in these situations? How do you handle situations in which acquaintances or strangers are not acting responsibly? What kinds of feedback do you usually give in these situations?

12. In what kinds of situations in your life do you feel the same kind of stress you felt during this activity? How can you apply what you learned in this activity about how you handle stress to those other situations?

13. What are some other situations in your life in which it is important to exercise self-control and self-discipline? How can you apply what you learned during this activity about your ability to exercise self-control and self-discipline to these situations?

14. Have you ever wanted to flip someone the bird? How did you feel in that situation? How did you handle that situation? If you did flip someone the bird, what happened? Was there something else you could have done to express your feelings that would have been a better way to handle the situation?

Safety Concerns: None, as long as participants are walking and watching for the bird.

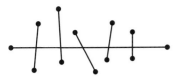 *I can do it with my left or my right—I'm almost amphibious! (whoops—ambidextrous)*

Name of Activity: Gotcha

Type of Activity: Icebreaker

Grade Level: Third grade and up

Size of Group: 5 to 200 (no kidding—works with 200)

Goal 2: Increase Self-Awareness and Self-Acceptance

Objectives:

2C. Develop ability to recognize negative self-talk
2D. Develop skills in replacing negative self-talk with positive self-talk

Goal 4: Increase Understanding and Valuing of Diversity

Objective:

4A. Recognize and appreciate individual differences

Goal 5: Demonstrate Consistently Responsible Behavior

Objectives:

5D. Develop coping skills for dealing with stress
5E. Understand the need for self-discipline and self-control and how to exercise them

Materials: None

Preparation: None

How to Play:

1. Have participants stand in a circle (or a rough equivalent of a circle for those circle-challenged groups), with members standing fairly close to one another (within easy reach).
2. Instruct participants to place their left hands, palms facing up, in front of the participant on their left. At this point, participants should be offering the palm of their left hands to the person on their left—and being offered the palm of a hand by the person on their right.
3. Instruct participants to extend their right index fingers and lift their right hands so they can place their right index fingers (pointing down) into the left hand being offered to them by the person on their right. At this point, all participants have their right index fingers dropping down into the left-hand palms of the participant on their right and have the right index finger of whoever is on their left placed in the palm of their left hands (easier to see than describe—try it—we think you'll get it).
4. Explain to the group that when you say "Gotcha!" the task is to capture the index finger in the palm of their left hand (by quickly closing their hand around the finger) while simultaneously avoiding the capture of their right index finger in the palm of their neighbor's left hand (by quickly lifting the finger out of their neighbor's hand before he or she can close his or her hand around it).
5. Repeat the directions slowly until you see that everyone has their right finger in the left palm of their neighbor and their neighbor's right finger in their left palm—then yell "GOTCHA!!" Note that at this point participants will try to grab their neighbor's finger in their left hand and, at the same time, quickly remove their finger from the hand of their neighbor.

Variations:

1. We like to use silly sound effects to place the finger in the palm of the hand like "wooooooo—Plop"—but then, that might just be us.

2. Noting that the person on your immediate left, whose finger you have in your left hand, is at a disadvantage (because you obviously know when you're going to say "Gotcha!"), instruct the group that this time the person to your immediate left will be the one to say the G word. Continue assigning leadership (who says the G-word) with each new round.

3. After participants get this down, switch hands. Have participants offer their right hands and place their left index fingers into the right hand of their neighbors. We suggest a different sound effect for the different hand.

4. As participants get better, invite them to place their left hand, palm down, out to their left about shoulder high. Instruct participants to place their right index fingers, point up now, into the right palm of their neighbors. Again, different sound effects may be required. Then switch hands again.

Sample Personalization-Processing Questions:

1. What was it like to wait for someone to say "Gotcha"?
2. How did it feel to be the one saying "Gotcha"?
3. What feelings did you experience as you were waiting for someone else to say "Gotcha"?
4. Who felt kind of stressed out as they were waiting?
5. Where did the stress come from?
6. Was it more or less stressful to be the one who was going to say "Gotcha" or the ones waiting for someone else to say it?
7. How did you deal with the stress of waiting?
8. Where did the stress manifest itself in your body?
9. How could someone just watching you play this game tell whether you were feeling anxious or stressed as you were waiting?
10. Did you feel as though you were successful at this game? What determined whether you felt successful?
11. Did you compare yourself to other members of the group when you were thinking about whether you were successful? How did that go for you?
12. What did you tell yourself about your ability to do this task as you were waiting?
13. What did you tell yourself about your ability to do this task the times when you weren't successful?
14. If you were using negative self-talk, how did this affect your ability to be successful?
15. If you were using positive self-talk, how did this affect your ability to be successful?
16. If you were using negative self-talk, how could you shift to more positive self-talk?
17. What strategies did you employ so that you could get better at catching and evading being caught?
18. Did you ever jump the gun by trying to catch or trying to get away from your neighbors before the leader said "Gotcha"? What was that about?
19. How did you work to gain the self-discipline and self-control to avoid jumping the gun?
20. How did you feel about making the silly noises?

Sample Application-Processing Questions:

1. As you were playing the game, did it feel really important that you avoided being caught by your neighbor and caught your neighbor's finger? In looking at your life, was it really important that you did those things? What do you think about the fact that it seemed important at the time, but might not have really been important?
2. What are some times in school when you get worried about something that turns out to not be a very big deal? At home?
3. How can you tell whether a situation is worth getting stressed out (or worried) about?
4. What are some of the ways that you let other people in your life know when you are feeling stressed or anxious?
5. How do you usually react when you are feeling stressed/anxious about a situation?
6. How do other people react to you when you are feeling stressed?
7. What do you usually do to cope with stressful situations? How do those coping strategies work for you?
8. What does it look like when you exercise self-discipline and self-control even though you are feeling stress?

9. Are there situations in your life in which negative self-talk might influence your ability to be successful? Positive self-talk?
10. What are some ways that you can shift negative self-talk into positive self-talk in those situations in which you are less successful that you could be due to negative self-talk?
11. Do you ever do things like make silly noises in public? If so, how do you feel when you do this? When would it be fun and when would it be embarrassing?
12. Does it change how embarrassing it is to do silly things when an entire group is participating in the silliness? If so, how does it change things?

Safety Concerns: None

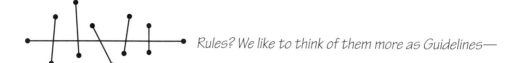

Name of Activity: Guidelines

Type of Activity: *Icebreaker; Deinhibitizer*

Grade Level: *Fourth grade and up*

Size of Group: *Up to about 100, depending on how much space you have (With more than 10 people, divide into smaller groups of 6 to 10 each.)*

Goal 1: Improve Communication and Relationship Skills

Objectives:

   1B.   Express feelings clearly and constructively
   1C.   Recognize and accept the feelings of others
   1D.   Express ideas clearly and constructively
   1E.   Listen actively to others
   1G.   Develop skills for making and maintaining relationships
   1H.   Recognize and deal with peer pressure
   1I.   Use communication skills to resolve conflict
   1L.   Develop skills for effectively participating in groups

Goal 2: Increase Self-Awareness and Self-Acceptance

Objectives:

   2A.   Explore personal attitudes and values
   2H.   Identify personal and social roles

Goal 4: Increase Understanding and Valuing of Diversity

Objectives:

   4A.   Recognize and appreciate individual differences
   4B.   Develop an understanding and appreciation of own culture
   4C.   Demonstrate respect for others as both individuals and members of different cultural groups
   4D.   Acknowledge and appreciate similarities and differences across cultures and/or groups of people who have physical or learning differences
   4E.   Recognize how stereotypes can affect interpersonal relationships and attitudes toward others

Materials: Open space; masking tape

Preparation: Using the masking tape, make a "course" for each subgroup. The course should consist of two parallel lines of tape that are about 12 feet long and 4 feet apart. Put a masking tape X in the middle of the opening at both ends of this course.

How to Play:

1.   Explain to the group members that this activity has only four rules that they must follow. Tell them:
   a.   The first rule is to not hurt yourself. Make sure that, as you do this activity, you keep yourself safe.
   b.   The second rule is that each of you must go from one X to another X three times. (This is an arbitrary number—you can have them go from one X to another X as many times as you

would like, depending on the amount of time you have, the size of your groups, and the group members' attention span. This activity shouldn't take more than about half an hour, though, so don't have a group of 10 do the between-the-X trip more than four or five times or it will take forever.)

    c. The third rule is that every trip you make from one X to another X should be unique, special, and different from every other trip by the other members of your group.

    d. The fourth rule is that when you successfully make it from one X to another X, the members of your group should acknowledge you in some way.

2. After giving them these directions, have them repeat the rules back to you to make sure that they have them clear in their minds and then let them have at it. (They are not going to like this—in most groups there are at least two or three members who want WAY more rules than this measly set. If they ask for clarification, just keep repeating the rules to them—with a smile of course—and if you want to look as if you know something that they don't know, that is totally up to you.)

3. After they have all finished the required number of repetitions, ask them to tell you again what the rules were. Then ask if anyone made up any other rules. Often, they will deny making up any rules, maybe even becoming indignant that you would be crass enough to suggest such a thing. (I certainly did the first time I played the game.) Eventually (perhaps with a little pump priming on your part as you begin to point out the rules you noticed them playing by) they will start admitting that, yes, they did make up a rule that they had to stay inside the parallel lines of tape; or they did make a rule that they had to use the Xs on their course rather than using some other group's Xs; or that they made up a rule that they all had to take turns, going one at a time; or that they all clapped to acknowledge one another's success, rather than some other form of acknowledgment, etc. Ask about what they felt/thought when someone in their group (or even in another group for those with wandering eyes) didn't follow one of the rules that they had made up.

4. You can then use this to help them look at all of the ways we make up rules in our everyday lives and challenge them to examine which of those rules are helpful to them and which of those rules get in their way. Point out that if someone else doesn't follow a rule that they had made up, there is a very good chance that it will irritate or upset them. Terry tells a story about when she was first married to her husband to illustrate the point. In Terry's family of origin, when they ate hotdogs, they always had yellow wax beans for a veggie. In Rick's family of origin, they always ate hotdogs with pork and beans. The first couple of years when they were married, they ate hotdogs a lot (they were poor, starving students) and had arguments about the proper thing to eat with hotdogs—they had different rules about hotdog companions. We are positive you can come up with your own examples in your life or in other interactions you have observed between group members. Wild and powerful discussions should ensue.[1]

Variations:

You can do this with a single individual: just have him or her make the X to another X journey five or six times.

Sample Personalization-Processing Questions:

1. What was your reaction when you first heard the directions for the game?
2. Did you follow all the rules laid out by the leader? Why or why not?
3. What was your reaction when the leader asked if anyone had made up any rules? How did you express your reaction to the leader and/or to the other members of the group?
4. What rules did you make up as you did the activity? How did you communicate about the rules you made up during the activity?
5. What rules made up by other people during the activity did you adapt as your own?
6. What was your reaction if other people violated one of the rules the leader had laid out? How did you express your feelings and thoughts in this situation?
7. What was your reaction if other people violated one of your rules? How did you express your feelings and thoughts in this situation?

---

[1]*Note.* Adapted from Beaudion, M., & Walden, S. (1998). *Working with groups to enhance relationships.* Duluth, MN: Whole Person Associates.

8. Did you experience peer pressure to conform to rules other people were following? How did you react when this happened? How did you communicate to other members of the group when this happened?

9. Did you exert peer pressure on others in the group to conform to your rules? How did you communicate that you thought they should be doing something differently? How did that work for you?

10. How were your family values and attitudes reflected in how you handled this activity? How were your cultural values and attitudes reflected in how you handled this activity?

11. How were the rules you made up different from the rules other members of the group made up? How were the rules you made up similar to the rules other members of the group made up?

12. Did you notice how other people reacted to your behavior during the game (i.e., if they approved or disapproved of what you were doing)? How did you feel if others approved of your behavior? How did you feel if others disapproved of your behavior? What did you do if you thought others approved of your behavior? What did you do if you thought others disapproved of your behavior?

13. Did you notice any patterns across the members in the group related to the rules people made up? What were those patterns? Were those patterns related in any way to the culture of those in the group?

14. Did you notice any stereotypes you were holding about certain people in this process? How did your holding those stereotypes affect how you interpreted what they did/the rules they made up?

15. If there were disagreements about rules among group members, how did you handle this? What were some ways you could have improved your ability to resolve any conflicts that occurred between group members?

16. Were there any patterns in whose rules got followed by other members of the group? Were there any patterns in whose rules got rejected by other members of the group? How was the relative status of people in the group reflected by these patterns?

Sample Application-Processing Questions:

1. Do you usually follow rules that are laid out by your family? By groups to which you belong? By society?

2. How do you decide which rules you are going to follow?

3. What are other situations or relationships in which you feel that you should stay between the lines? What are situations or relationships in which you give yourself permission to step out of the lines? What determines which reaction you have?

4. What are some rules that you have made up in your life?

5. What are some rules made up by your family that you act as if they must be followed? Friends? Your culture? Society? Other groups? How can you apply what you learned in this activity to deal more effectively with those situations?

6. How can you go about detecting these hidden rules in your life? In your relationships?

7. How do you decide whether these rules are serving you any longer?

8. Which of these rules work well for you?

9. Which of the rules you made up are no longer serving you?

10. Which of the rules made up by others are no longer serving you?

11. What do you want to do about the rules that are no longer serving you?

12. As you look at your life as compared to other people (i.e., in your school, in your family, in your work, in your church, in your culture, in society, etc.), do you have more or fewer rules than others? Is your adherence to your rules more strict or less strict than others? How do your rules about rules affect the way you live your life?

13. How do you feel when you are not following one of your own rules? What do you do about these feelings? How can you apply what you learned in this activity to deal more effectively with those situations?

14. How do you feel when you are not following one of the rules made up by others? What happens in your life when this happens? How can you apply what you learned in this activity to deal more effectively with those situations?

15. How do you feel when someone is not following one of your rules? What do you do about it when this happens? How can you apply what you learned in this activity to deal more effectively with those situations?
16. What happens in a situation in which someone has a rule that he or she hasn't told to the other people involved? Does this ever happen with you? How do you react in these situations? How can you apply what you learned in this activity to deal more effectively with those situations?
17. How would clear and constructive communication be helpful in these situations?
18. How can you cultivate becoming more respectful to others when they are living by different rules than you are?

Safety Concerns: None, as long as they follow the first rule, which was to keep themselves safe when on their journey.

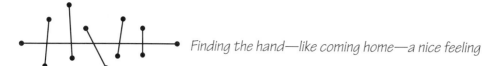
Finding the hand—like coming home—a nice feeling

Name of Activity: Hand Find

Type of Activity: *Icebreaker; Trust*

Grade Level: *First grade and up*

Size of Group: *2 to 30 (more if you have the space and some folks who will help you herd participants back to the group if they start to wander off)*

Goal 1: Improve Communication and Relationship Skills

Objectives:

1F.   Demonstrate willingness to trust others
1G.   Develop skills for making and maintaining relationships

Goal 2: Increase Self-Awareness and Self-Acceptance

Objectives:

2C.   Develop ability to recognize negative self-talk
2D.   Develop skills in replacing negative self-talk with positive self-talk
2E.   Appreciate own uniqueness
2G.   Recognize personal boundaries, rights, and privacy needs

Goal 4: Increase Understanding and Valuing of Diversity

Objectives:

4A.   Recognize and appreciate individual differences
4B.   Develop an understanding and appreciation of own culture
4C.   Demonstrate respect for others as both individuals and members of different cultural groups
4D.   Acknowledge and appreciate similarities and differences across cultures and/or groups of people who have physical or learning differences

Goal 5: Demonstrate Consistently Responsible Behavior

Objectives:

5A.   Acknowledge personal responsibilities
5B.   Recognize whether behavior is appropriate and responsible
5C.   Act in an appropriate and responsible manner
5D.   Develop coping skills for dealing with stress
5E.   Understand the need for self-discipline and self-control and how to exercise them

Goal 6: Enhance Positive Attitudes and Skills Related to Learning

Objectives:

6A.   Develop feeling of competence and confidence as a learner
6B.   Take pride in accomplishments
6C.   Accept mistakes as part of the learning process
6E.   Recognize that effort and persistence enhance learning
6H.   Develop critical-thinking skills

Materials: Open space; you may decide that you want blindfolds if you want to really make sure folks do the activity "blind," and you don't think you can trust them to keep their eyes closed (though this may limit your numbers—I don't know about you, but we don't carry 100 blindfolds around just in case we need them).

Preparation: If you have a wide open space or things that might trip participants if they wandered too far off or hard walls, you may want to solicit several helpers to herd participants who are meandering off from the group back to the fold.

How to Play:

1. Have the participants divide into pairs, and introduce themselves if they don't already know one another.
2. We like to tell the group that each person is a unique and special person, different from all others. As one way to help them really "get" this, you are going to ask them to get to know one another in a physical way, by exploring one another's hands. In order to do this, they will take turns touching their partner's hands, noticing how big the hands are, how long the fingers are, how thick the knuckles are, how the fingernails feel, and so forth. The idea is that they could recognize their partner's hands by touch.
3. After a certain amount of time (depending on the group and their maturity, they may really get into this exploration, so give them an appropriate amount of time), ask them to mill about the room, moving away from their partner. After about a minute or two of this, ask them to close their eyes (or put on their blindfolds, depending on how much you trust the group to close their eyes) and continue to mill about for a while.
4. After moment or two of blind milling about (to make sure they have no idea where their partner is now), ask them to put their hands out, touch the hands of the people they encounter and find their partner by touch alone.
5. As they slowly walk about the space, touching one another's hands, they may wander off from the group. This should activate the herders' sheep dog instincts, and the wanderers should be gently guided back to the main group.
6. When the first pair or two finds one another, let them know that they might want to move to the side so that they don't get in the way of the folks who are still questing for their partners.

Variations:

1. You can ask them to become acquainted in more than one way simultaneously. As they learn one another's hands, they can also talk about themselves and their likes and dislikes, positive qualities, things that are challenging for them, things that make them unique, etc.
2. Once they get the hang of this, if you want them to make a close connection with more than one person, you can ask them to find a different partner and do it again.
3. If you have a really "advanced" group, you can even do this with more than two people at a time; so have a group of three, four, or five learn one another's hands and find one another in the crowd.

Sample Personalization-Processing Questions:

1. As your partner was learning your hand, what did you notice about your own hand?
2. As you felt the different hands, what did you notice about the hands? Were they all the same? Were they all unique?
3. How did you feel about wandering around in a group of people touching one another with their eyes closed?
4. How did you make sure that you did not get touched in a way that was uncomfortable to you? If someone did touch you in a way that was uncomfortable for you, what did you do about it?
5. Did you keep your eyes closed the entire activity? How did your level of trust of the group influence whether or not you chose to keep your eyes closed? How did your level of trust for yourself and your ability to find your partner influence whether or not you chose to keep your eyes closed?
6. What method did you use to help you remember what your partner's hand felt like? What was your strategy for finding your partner?
7. If you were one of the folks who took a longer time to find your partner, what were you telling yourself about your ability to find your partner? How did your thoughts about your abilities (either negative self-talk or positive self-talk) affect the likelihood of your finding your partner? If you were feeling discouraged, what strategies did you use to keep yourself going and not give up?

8. If you thought you had found your partner and discovered that you had made a mistake and claimed someone else, how did you feel about making that mistake? What did you tell yourself about making a mistake? If you had negative thoughts about yourself and your abilities, what did you do about those thoughts? How could you have gone about changing any negative self-talk into more positive self-talk?

9. If you started wandering away from the group and had to be herded back, how did you feel about it? Did you think you had made a mistake? What did you tell yourself about making a mistake? If you had negative thoughts about yourself and your abilities, what did you do about those thoughts? How could you have gone about changing any negative self-talk into more positive self-talk?

10. If you originally claimed the wrong person, how did you revise your strategies when you went back to searching for your partner?

11. How did you feel when you finally found your partner?

12. What were your responsibilities to the group in this activity? How did you decide what your responsibilities were?

13. Did you honor those responsibilities in playing this activity? If yes, what kinds of things did you do that you felt were responsible? How did you make sure your behavior was responsible? If no, what kinds of things did you do that you felt were not responsible? What kept you from being responsible during this activity?

14. What about this activity made it important to exercise self-discipline and self-control?

15. What did you find stressful in this activity? What strategies did you use to cope with this stress?

Sample Application-Processing Questions:

1. In other situations in your life, how comfortable are you with physical touch? How much do you have to trust someone to touch them? Allow them to touch you?

2. What are some other situations in your life in which you feel as if you are blindly searching for something or someone? How do you feel about those situations? How do you handle those situations?

3. How do you usually decide whether to trust or not trust? How are your behaviors and reactions different in situations in which you are trusting versus situations in which you are not trusting?

4. What could you learn from this game that you could apply in situations in which it would be important to recognize and maintain your personal boundaries, rights, and privacy needs?

5. What are the rules (spoken or unspoken) about physical touch and/or physical closeness in your family? In your culture?

6. What are some other situations in which you have noticed differences in people's comfort levels about physical touch and/or physical closeness? What were the differences that you noticed?

7. What have you noticed about different cultural groups and their rules about physical touch and/or physical closeness?

8. If someone else has different rules than you do about physical touch and/or physical closeness, how can you handle this in an appropriate, respectful way?

9. What are some situations or relationships in which you feel that it is really important to act in a responsible manner? How do you handle these situations or relationships?

10. What are some times when you do not act as responsibly as you think you should? What do you think keeps you from being responsible in those situations? How could you handle those situations differently in the future?

11. How do you feel when you get feedback that you are not acting in a responsible manner? How do you react to this feedback? How is your reaction affected by who it is that is giving the feedback?

12. In what kinds of situations in your life do you feel the same kind of stress you felt during this activity? How can you apply what you learned about how you handle stress in this activity to those other situations?

13. What are some other situations in your life in which it is important to exercise self-control and self-discipline? How can you apply what you learned during this activity about your ability to exercise self-control and self-discipline to these situations?

14. What are some other situations in your life in which a person's willingness to act in a responsible manner can affect your ability to trust him or her?

15. How do you usually handle situations in which you are not immediately successful? When you are successful at something that was difficult for you, how do you usually feel? How do you handle those situations?

16. What do you usually tell yourself about yourself or your abilities when you make a mistake or are not immediately successful at something? What are some other situations or relationships in which you might be telling yourself negative things about yourself or your abilities? How do you feel in these situations or relationships? What are some strategies you have used for shifting your self-talk in a more positive direction?

17. What are some other situations in your life in which you could notice and celebrate your own uniqueness? Your successes?

Safety Concerns: Make sure folks don't wander off blindly, hit walls, or trip over obstacles. This is why you have those herders to help you if the crowd is large.

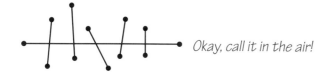
Okay, call it in the air!

Name of Activity: Heads or Tails

Type of Activity: *Icebreaker; Deinhibitizer*

Grade Level: *First grade and up*

Size of Group: *8 to 100 (crazy with 100—but fun)*

Goal 2: Increase Self-Awareness and Self-Acceptance
Objective:

2H.   Identify personal and social roles

Goal 3: Develop and Apply Problem-Solving and Decision-Making Skills
Objectives:

3D.   Evaluate decisions
3E.   Manage change and transitions in everyday life
3G.   Apply decision-making skills in life situations
3H.   Demonstrate effective coping skills for dealing with problems
3I.   Recognize when peer pressure is influencing decision making
3J.   Develop ability to identify alternative methods for solving problems and achieving goals

Goal 5: Demonstrate Consistently Responsible Behavior
Objectives:

5B.   Recognize whether behavior is appropriate and responsible
5C.   Act in an appropriate and responsible manner
5D.   Develop coping skills for dealing with stress
5E.   Understand the need for self-discipline and self-control and how to exercise them

Materials: Something to flip in order to indicate heads or tails. You can obviously use a coin. For fun we often use something large (and often silly) to flip. Anything with two distinct sides will work. You might try a large frisbee, a large block of wood painted two different colors, etc.

Preparation: Set up boundaries for the activity to take place in. The activity can take place in a large or small space depending on the number of participants and whether you instruct them to run, walk, or walk in slow motion.

How to Play:

1.   In this activity the heads or tails chase each other depending upon the flip of a coin (or object).
2.   Have the participants gather in a large circle with some space between each participant.
3.   Tell participants that on the count of three they will be asked to declare either heads or tails by placing their hands either on the top of their heads (indicating heads) or on their tails (i.e., behind; indicating tails).
4.   Explain to participants that the flip of a coin (or object) will decide whether the heads or the tails are It in the game. For example, if the coin (or object) comes up heads, then heads are It.
5.   Once each player has declared either heads or tails, the leader in the middle flips the coin or object.
6.   If the coin or object lands with the heads side up, the people with their hands on their heads are It and must chase the people with the hands on their tails around the room.
7.   Note that participants must have one hand on either their head or tail throughout each round of the activity.

8. Once tagged, a tails person moves his or her hand from his or her tail to his or her head and helps the heads chase the tails until everyone becomes a head.
9. If the coin/object lands tails up, then the tails are It, and the process is the same with the heads becoming tails and helping catch the other heads.
10. Once everyone has been tagged, participants return to the circle to begin another round. Play can continue for as many rounds as participants want to play (typically three to four rounds).[1]

Variations:

One variation we sometimes use is that those who are tagged (e.g., the heads who are tagged by the tails) join hands with the ones who tagged them. Their new pursuit of other tails has to happen while holding hands. Typically, at the end each of the heads (or whichever side was It) is holding the hands of at least one former tails.

Sample Personalization-Processing Questions:

1. How did you decide whether to be a head or a tail each time? Did you look around to see whether other people were choosing to be heads or tails? How did the other people and their choices influence your choosing?
2. How did the transitions (when you were tagged and had to switch from being a taggee to a tagger) go for you?
3. When you were a taggee, how did you feel when you got caught by the tagger? When you were the tagger, how did you feel when you caught the taggee?
4. Which role did you like best (taggee or tagger)? What did you like about it? What did you dislike about the other role?
5. What were your responsibilities to the group in this activity? How did you decide what your responsibilities were?
6. Did you honor those responsibilities in playing this activity? If yes, what kinds of things did you do that you felt were responsible? How did you make sure your behavior was responsible? If no, what kinds of things did you do that you felt were not responsible? What kept you from being responsible during this activity?
7. How could you tell whether other people perceived your behaviors as responsible? What kinds of feedback did you get from others about whether you were being responsible during this activity? How did you react when you got this feedback?
8. Did you feel that the other members of the group were acting responsibly during these activities? What kind of feedback did you give others about their acting responsibly during this activity?
9. What about this activity made it important to exercise self-discipline and self-control? How did you do with self-discipline and self-control?
10. On a 1 to 10 scale, what was your stress level during this activity? Did your stress level change depending on whether you were the taggee or the tagger? What did you find stressful in this activity? What made that stressful? What strategies did you use to cope with this stress?

Sample Application-Processing Questions:

1. In relationships with friends and family members, are you more comfortable as the pursuer or the pursued? What do you like about that role? How often do you play that role in relationships?
2. How often do you play the other role? What is uncomfortable for you about that role?
3. Are there other roles you play in your relationships (besides pursuer or pursued)? What are they? How often do you play these roles? How comfortable are you in each of these roles?
4. Have you observed other members of your family or your friends playing the role of pursuer or pursued? How do you feel about this when it happens?
5. What are some other situations in which you are sometimes influenced by what others do, say, or think? When is that a constructive approach to making a decision? When is that a self-defeating way to make a decision? How would you like to do this differently?
6. What are some situations or relationships when you feel that it is really important to act in a responsible manner? How do you handle these situations or relationships?

[1] *Note.* Adapted from Rohnke, K., & Butler, S. (1995). *Quicksilver.* Dubuque, IA: Kendall Hunt.

7. What are some times when you do not act as responsibly as you think you should? What do you think keeps you from being responsible in those situations? How could you handle those situations differently in the future?

8. How do you feel when you get feedback that you are not acting in a responsible manner? How do you react to this feedback? How is your reaction affected by who it is that is giving the feedback?

9. How do you handle situations in which friends or family members are not acting responsibly? What kinds of feedback do you usually give in these situations? How do you handle situations in which acquaintances or strangers are not acting responsibly? What kinds of feedback do you usually give in these situations?

10. In what kinds of situations in your life do you feel the same kind of stress you felt during this activity? How can you apply what you learned about how you handle stress during this activity to those other situations?

11. What are some other situations in your life in which it is important to exercise self-control and self-discipline? How can you apply what you learned during this activity about your ability to exercise self-control and self-discipline to these situations?

12. How do you usually handle transitions from one role to another? What are some things you like about how you handle these transitions? What are some things you don't like about how you handle these transitions? How could you get better at handling transitions from one role to another?

Safety Concerns: We always recommend walking of some variation for safety. You may also want to consider playing on a soft surface as participants can jostle one another.

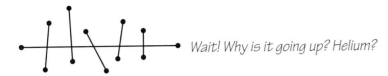
Wait! Why is it going up? Helium?

Name of Activity: Helium Stick

Type of Activity: Challenge/Initiative

Grade Level: Fifth grade and up

Size of Group: 10 to 20

Goal 1: Improve Communication and Relationship Skills

Objectives:

1A.   Demonstrate understanding of and apply basic communication skills (e.g., recognizing nonverbal cues, delivering "I" messages)
1B.   Express feelings clearly and constructively
1C.   Recognize and accept the feelings of others
1D.   Express ideas clearly and constructively
1E.   Listen actively to others
1F.   Demonstrate willingness to trust others
1G.   Develop skills for making and maintaining relationships
1H.   Recognize and deal with peer pressure
1I.   Use communication skills to resolve conflict
1J.   Recognize the need for help and develop the ability to ask for it
1K.   Recognize and verbalize needs and wishes
1L.   Develop skills for effectively participating in groups

Goal 2: Increase Self-Awareness and Self-Acceptance

Objectives:

2C.   Develop ability to recognize negative self-talk
2D.   Develop skills in replacing negative self-talk with positive self-talk
2F.   Develop positive attitudes toward self
2G.   Recognize personal boundaries, rights, and privacy needs
2H.   Identify personal and social roles

Goal 3: Develop and Apply Problem-Solving and Decision-Making Skills

Objectives:

3A.   Set personal goals
3B.   Identify problems
3C.   Demonstrate understanding of steps for solving problems and making decisions (gather information; explore alternatives and consequences; plan and take action)
3D.   Evaluate decisions
3F.   Apply decision-making skills to resolve conflicts
3H.   Demonstrate effective coping skills for dealing with problems
3I.   Recognize when peer pressure is influencing decision making
3J.   Develop ability to identify alternative methods for solving problems and achieving goals

Goal 5: Demonstrate Consistently Responsible Behavior

Objectives:

5A.   Acknowledge personal responsibilities
5B.   Recognize whether behavior is appropriate and responsible

5C. Act in an appropriate and responsible manner
5D. Develop coping skills for dealing with stress
5E. Understand the need for self-discipline and self-control and how to exercise them
5G. Demonstrate respect for alternate perspectives

Goal 6: Enhance Positive Attitudes and Skills Related to Learning

Objectives:

6C. Accept mistakes as part of the learning process
6G. Develop the ability to share knowledge
6H. Develop critical-thinking skills

Materials: We usually use a long tent pole, but any long, relatively thin, and very light object would work (e.g., a long broomstick or rake handle). The object needs to be long enough to get at least 10 people to hold it (i.e., two groups of 5 people, each group of 5 standing shoulder to shoulder with the two groups of 5 facing each other).

Preparation: Prepare yourself not to snicker when the helium stick goes up instead of down.

How to Play:

1. Have the group split up into two roughly equal subgroups (if 10 total then 5 on a side, if 11 then 5 on one side and 6 on the other).
2. Have each subgroup stand shoulder to shoulder (side by side) facing the other subgroup standing roughly 3 feet apart. At this point, there will be 5 people (in the case of 10 total) standing side by side facing 5 other people who are also standing side by side.
3. Have all of the participants raise both hands to roughly shoulder level and point at the line of people across from them. Explain to the group that the object of the activity is to allow the tent pole to rest on their fingers and, as a group, simply lower the tent pole to the ground.
4. After explaining the rules carefully (emphasizing the "simply lower it to the ground" part), we place the tent pole on the group members' fingers, carefully keeping hold of it. To do this, we often sneak between a couple of the people in one of the lines facing the other line. There is typically some jostling here as people move a little forward or adjust themselves side to side so that all can get their fingers under the tent pole.
5. Further explain that participants should not change the posture of their pointing fingers (keep them parallel to the ground), should keep their thumbs out of the way (simply let the tent pole rest on their fingers), and should not let their fingers break contact with the tent pole (let it rest on their fingers and lower it to the ground).
6. Continuing to hold the tent pole, remind participants of the rules, "Don't change the angle of your fingers (keep them parallel to the ground), let the tent pole rest on your fingers, don't break contact with the tent pole, simply lower it to the ground." At this point you will likely feel pressure UP on the tent pole (as the group attempts to make sure they don't lose contact).
7. Say "Go" and let go of the tent pole.
8. Although it might not happen immediately, nearly every time we do the activity (with at least 10 people) the tent pole goes up rather than down (hence the name Helium Stick).
9. We love to say, after the tent pole has gone up (sometimes higher than some participants can reach), "Okay, let's review," and then repeat the rules.
10. The tendency for participants, when the tent pole starts to rise, is to let the tent pole rise above their fingers (sometimes to show "it's not me, it's not my fault the pole is rising instead of falling"). When participants do this, or you think they are about to, we like to remind them, "Please don't stop making contact." Similarly, if the tent pole does not go down right away, it is likely that some participants will try to lower their hands to start the pole down and will break contact. When they do so, we also like to remind them, "Please don't break contact."
11. This is a great activity to show that working together is actually deceptively easy (hence, our fun with the directive to "simply lower the tent pole").

Variations:

To save time, we will sometimes interrupt the activity and choose two participants (especially if there are two who have been scapegoated or blamed in initial processing) to complete the same task. Tell them, "Stand facing each other; point at the other person; let the tent pole rest on your fingers; don't change the angle of your fingers; don't break contact with the tent pole; simply lower it to the ground." Two participants can complete the task easily, making for an interesting comparison and interesting discussion.

Sample Personalization-Processing Questions:

1. What was your initial reaction to the instructions? What was your reaction to the instructions as they were repeated several times as the tent pole went up instead of down?
2. How did you feel as it became clear that this task was not as easy as it initially sounded? How did you express your feelings to the rest of the group? How could you have expressed your feelings more clearly and constructively?
3. How did the other members of the group feel as it became clear that this task was not as easy as it initially sounded? How did they express their feelings to the rest of the group? How could they have expressed their feelings more clearly and constructively?
4. What did the general frustration inherent in this process do to the group dynamics?
5. What was your reaction to the seeming impossibility of lowering the tent pole to the ground?
6. Did your group try to develop strategies so that you could be more successful? How did you go about developing those strategies?
7. Did everyone feel heard as the group tried to develop strategies for lowering the tent pole to the ground? How did it feel when you were heard by other members of the group? What did you do to try to make sure that you were heard by the other members of the group?
8. If you didn't feel heard, what was that like for you? If you had wanted to be heard by the other members of the group, what could you have done differently to make sure that you were heard?
9. Did you communicate your ideas and feelings effectively? If so, how did you go about doing this? If not, what prevented you from doing this?
10. If your strategy for lowering the tent pole to the ground was not working, what did the members of the group do? Did you blame one another? If yes, how did people react to this? If no, (congratulations—you are a rare breed!), how did you avoid this common occurrence?
11. How did the members of the group go about developing an alternative strategy when it became apparent that a strategy wasn't working?
12. How could you tell whether you needed help from other group members? What did you do when you needed help? How did you ask for help when you recognized you needed it? What impact did helping one another have on the process?
13. What roles did various group members play in the process of lowering the pole to the ground? Did leaders and followers emerge? If so, how did the group members work out who was going to lead and who was going to follow? If no leaders emerged, how did that go for the group?
14. If your group was not successful at lowering the pole to the ground, how did this affect the leadership? Did the roles change during the course of the activity as a result of the stress of not being able to lower the pole?
15. How did you feel about being physically close and/or touching one another as you held the pole? How much personal space do you need? How is this different from the other people in the group and their personal space requirements?
16. If you were one of the people who was blamed for messing up, how did you feel about this? What did you tell yourself about your competence when this happened? What did you tell yourself about other group members when this happened? What did you communicate to the rest of the group when messing up happened?
17. If you were one of the people who felt you were not messing up when others were, how did you feel about this? How did you express your feelings to the group? How could you have expressed these feelings in a clearer and more constructive way?
18. What was your level of stress during this activity? How did it change as time passed? If you had a time limit, how did this affect your stress level? What strategies did you use to cope with the stress involved in this activity? Which of these strategies were effective? Which were not? Why?

19. When members of the group disagreed on strategies for lowering the pole, how did you feel about the disagreement? What did you do about your feelings? Did the disagreement escalate into a conflict? How did the group members resolve the conflict? What would have been some other (better?) ways to do this?

20. In what ways did peer pressure affect the process? How did the members of your group handle the peer pressure?

21. What personal positive traits and talents did you bring to this process, and how did you use them to help in getting everyone through the experience?

22. If you were feeling discouraged in this process, how did you deal with that? What did you tell yourself to motivate yourself to continue? If other group members were feeling discouraged, how did you interact with them about their discouragement?

23. How did you feel about it if the group actually lowered the pole to the ground? How did you communicate those feelings to the rest of the group?

24. What were your responsibilities to the group in this activity? How did you decide what your responsibilities were?

25. Did you act in a responsible way during this activity? If yes, how did you act in a responsible way? How did you make sure your behavior was responsible? If no, how did you act in an irresponsible way? What kept you from acting more responsibly?

26. Why was acting with self-discipline and self-control important in this activity?

27. If your group did the activity as a large group and then as a small group, what was the difference between the two experiences? Why was it easier for the smaller group to follow the directions?

Sample Application-Processing Questions:

1. Have you ever been in a situation that seemed impossible to master? How did you handle that situation? What did you learn from this activity that you could apply in those situations in the future? When you are in situations that seem impossible to master, what resources do you have to help you deal with these situations?

2. Have you ever been in a relationship in which the parties blame one another for things when they do not go the way they should? How have you handled those relationships in the past? What did you learn from this activity that you could apply in those relationships in the future?

3. When you are in situations that are very challenging for you, what do you usually tell yourself about yourself and your abilities? How can you improve your ability to use positive self-talk in those situations?

4. How do you define success in other situations in your life? How can you apply what you learned in this activity about yourself and the way you think and feel about success to other situations in your life?

5. What happens for you when you are in a group that is not being successful in the tasks it is attempting? How can you be more positive and proactive in these situations?

6. How did the role(s) you played in this group resemble your role(s) in your family? In other groups? How do the other roles taken by various group members resemble roles taken by the other people in your life? What is your comfort level about these roles?

7. Which of the methods for managing stress that you or the members of your group used could be helpful in other situations in your life? How can you use them on a more regular basis?

8. What are some other situations in which you might need to ask for help? How can you get better about recognizing when you need help and asking for it?

9. What are some other situations or relationships in which it might be important for you to be heard? How can you go about making sure that you are heard in those situations?

10. How can you apply some of the methods for communicating about feelings and ideas, encouraging cooperation, solving problems, and/or appropriately resolving conflicts that became evident in this activity?

11. How can you apply what you learned about dealing with mistakes in other situations? Dealing with negative self-talk? Encouraging persistence and flexibility? Dealing with peer pressure?

12. What could you learn from this game that you could apply in situations in which it would be important to recognize and maintain your personal boundaries, rights, and privacy needs?

13. What are the rules (spoken or unspoken) about personal space and/or touching in your family? In your culture?
14. If someone else has different rules than you do about personal space, how can you handle this in an appropriate and respectful way?
15. What did you learn about your critical-thinking skills that you can apply to other situations in your life?
16. What are some other situations in your life in which you could notice and celebrate your talents, abilities, contributions? Your successes?
17. What are the rules about getting it right in your family? What are your rules about getting it right? Are there some of those rules that have a negative impact on you when you don't get it right? How could you change your rules about getting it right?
18. How do you usually handle situations in which you are not in control of whether something works out or not? What did you learn from your experience in this activity that you can use to help you handle those situations better?
19. How do you usually handle situations in which you are not able to live up to your own standards? What did you learn from your experience in this activity that you can use to help you handle those situations better?

Safety Concerns: None except for the tendency for frustrated participants to turn on each other.

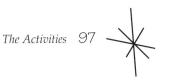

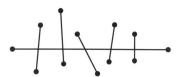 *Focusing on the things that hold us together!*

Name of Activity: Holding It All Together

Type of Activity: *Challenge/Initiative*

Grade Level: *Third grade and up*

Size of Group: *4 to 15*

Goal 1: Improve Communication and Relationship Skills

Objectives:

- 1A. Demonstrate understanding of and apply basic communication skills (e.g., recognizing nonverbal cues, delivering "I" messages)
- 1D. Express ideas clearly and constructively
- 1E. Listen actively to others
- 1G. Develop skills for making and maintaining relationships
- 1H. Recognize and deal with peer pressure
- 1I. Use communication skills to resolve conflict
- 1J. Recognize the need for help and develop the ability to ask for it
- 1K. Recognize and verbalize needs and wishes
- 1L. Develop skills for effectively participating in groups

Goal 2: Increase Self-Awareness and Self-Acceptance

Objective:

- 2A. Explore personal attitudes and values

Goal 3: Develop and Apply Problem-Solving and Decision-Making Skills

Objectives:

- 3C. Demonstrate understanding of steps for solving problems and making decisions (gather information; explore alternatives and consequences; plan and take action)
- 3D. Evaluate decisions
- 3E. Manage change and transitions in everyday life
- 3F. Apply decision-making skills to resolve conflicts
- 3G. Apply decision-making skills in life situations
- 3H. Demonstrate effective coping skills for dealing with problems
- 3I. Recognize when peer pressure is influencing decision making
- 3J. Develop ability to identify alternative methods for solving problems and achieving goals

Goal 4: Increase Understanding and Valuing of Diversity (if using variation # 4)

Objectives:

- 4A. Recognize and appreciate individual differences
- 4C. Demonstrate respect for others as both individuals and members of different cultural groups
- 4D. Acknowledge and appreciate similarities and differences across cultures and/or groups of people who have physical or learning differences

Goal 6: Enhance Positive Attitudes and Skills Related to Learning (if using Variation 3)

Objectives:

- 6A. Develop feeling of competence and confidence as a learner
- 6E. Recognize that effort and persistence enhance learning

6G.   Develop the ability to share knowledge
6H.   Develop critical-thinking skills

Materials: Five to six short pieces of rope or cords about 10 feet long. If ropes are all one length and/or color it makes the task more difficult; if ropes are different lengths/colors the task is easier.

Preparation: Tie all but one of the ropes into loops or circles (e.g., tie the two ends of the ropes to each other with a simple knot like a square knot). Pass the last rope through all of the other loops and then knot this last rope into a loop. Arrange this collection of connected loops out on the ground so that the single encompassing loop is not necessarily obvious.

How to Play:

1.   Gather the group around the ropes.
2.   Ask the group to examine the five loops of rope on the ground and come to consensus on which rope loop holds all the rest of the ropes or cords together. Sometimes we have groups vote, rather than work to come to consensus, on the rope they think holds the rest.
3.   Explain to the group that they cannot move, touch, untangle, or unravel any of the ropes or knots.
4.   After the group has reached consensus (or voted) have one of participants pick up the rope the group has identified as holding all the rest—and let the group see if they are right!![1]

Variations:

1.   This activity often works best if you start with five different color ropes. After the group has completed the task, move to a more difficult scenario in which all the ropes are the exact same color or pattern.
2.   With an older group (fifth grade and up), you can have the participants identify five or six values or characteristics that are important to the group and write them down (these often include things like honesty, integrity, support, etc.). We often then have a discussion about which of these (or some other) is the main or overarching value or characteristic that really connects or holds together the rest of the values or characteristics. Then say to the group, "The five ropes in front of you represent the values of the group. There is also an overarching value that connects all the other values together. Your task is to find that overarching value without touching anything." What great practice for the group to look for that main value!
3.   Using a different metaphor, you can frame the loops as a big problem (collection of loops) made up from a number of little problems (each knotted loop). You can tell the group, "As is often the case with big problems, solving the initial crux problem often leads to solving the rest of the problem. Without actually touching the problem in any way, your task is to discover and agree on which of the problems is holding the entire problem together."
4.   Using a different metaphor, you can frame the loops as different kinds of people. You can use ethnic or cultural groups, different kinds of learners, people of different ages, etc. Then have the group members describe more specifically the characteristics of all five of the different kinds of people. Then ask the group to generate a list of qualities that all of the people they are describing have in common. When they have done this, tell them that you want them to find the loop "holding them all together just like those qualities they all share," without touching any of the ropes or knots.

Sample Personalization-Processing Questions:

1.   What was your reaction when you first heard the directions to this activity? How did you express your thoughts and feelings? Did your reaction change as the group discussed strategies? How?
2.   What did you do to contribute to the success of the group? How did you feel about your contribution?
3.   Did you feel heard as the group members worked on solving the problem? How did it feel when you were heard by other members of the group?

[1]*Note.* Adapted from Cain, J., & Jolliff, B. (1998). *Teamwork and teamplay.* Dubuque, IA: Kendall Hunt and Priest, S., & Rohnke, K. (1999). *101 of the best corporate team-building activities we know.* Dubuque, IA: Kendall Hunt.

4. If you didn't feel heard, what was that like for you? If you had wanted to be heard by the other members of the group, what could you have done differently to make sure that you were heard?
5. Did you communicate your ideas and feelings effectively? If so, how did you go about doing this? If not, what prevented you from doing this?
6. What did you do in your role as a listener to make the process in this activity go more smoothly?
7. What process did the members of the group use to determine which rope was holding it all together? How did the group come to a consensus?
8. How did you feel if (when?) your group guessed wrong? How did you express those feelings to other members of the group?
9. When members of the group struggled with coming to consensus, did it feel like conflict to you? How did you feel about the conflict? What did you do about your feelings? How did the group members resolve the conflict? What would have been some other ways to do this?
10. In what ways did peer pressure affect the process? How did the members of your group handle the peer pressure?
11. If you were feeling stressed and/or discouraged in this process, how did you deal with that? What did you tell yourself to motivate yourself to continue? If other group members were feeling stressed and/or discouraged, how did you interact with them about their feelings? How could you have been more supportive?
12. How did you feel about it when the group guessed which rope was holding it all together correctly? How did you communicate those feelings to the rest of the group?
13. What role did persistence play in the group's success or failure at this activity?
14. If your initial guess was incorrect, how did the group members use what they had learned from this failure to increase their chances of successfully guessing in subsequent tries?
15. What values are most important to you? How do you communicate about those values to others? How do you handle it when other people do not share your values?
16. How did the members of your group identify five or six values or characteristics that were important to the group? How did you choose the overarching value or characteristic that linked them? Did you agree with the values or characteristics the group chose? If you didn't, how did you react/communicate to the group about your lack of agreement? (Variation 2)
17. How did the members of your group choose the different kinds of people? What were the characteristics the group members chose to describe each group? How did the members of the group decide what all of the people you were describing had in common? Did you agree with the characteristics the group chose? If you didn't, how did you react/communicate to the group about your lack of agreement? (Variation 4)

Sample Application-Processing Questions:

1. How do you feel about the process of reaching consensus?
2. What are other situations or relationships in your life in which reaching consensus is important? How can you apply what you learned in this activity about reaching consensus in these situations?
3. How do you go about solving problems that are similar to the problem that needed to be solved in this activity? Which of the methods for problem solving used by the members of your group would be useful in other situations in your life? How can you use them in these situations?
4. What are some other situations or relationships in which it is important for you to be heard? How can you go about making sure that you are heard in those situations?
5. What are some other situations or relationships in which it might be important for you to use effective listening skills? How can you go about making sure that you are using effective listening skills in those situations?
6. How can you apply some of the methods for communicating about feelings and ideas, encouraging cooperation, solving problems, persistence, and/or appropriately resolving conflicts that you learned/practiced in this activity in other situations?
7. What are some other situations in which you have noticed similarities and differences across different groups of people? What were the similarities that you noticed? What are the differences you have noticed? How can you acknowledge and celebrate these commonalities and differences in a respectful way?

8. How do you deal with situations in which you disagree with what the other members of a group decide? How can you apply what you learned in this activity to those situations?

9. What did you learn about your critical-thinking skills that you can apply to other situations in your life?

10. Why is it important to know what your own attitudes and values are? What are some situations in your life in which it is critical to be really clear about your own attitudes and values?

11. What are some situations in your life in which it is critical to share your knowledge with others? How do you feel when you get to share your knowledge with others?

12. How can you apply some of the methods that you learned/practiced in this activity for dealing with peer pressure, handling stress, asking for help, and/or handling transitions in other situations?

Safety Concerns: None

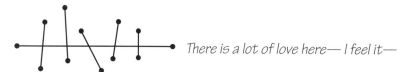
There is a lot of love here— I feel it—

Name of Activity: Hug Tag

Type of Activity: Deinhibitizer

Grade Level: First grade and up

Size of Group: 8 to 100, maybe more

Goals: You mean, besides making the facilitator/leader laugh out loud?

Goal 1: Improve Communication and Relationship Skills

Objectives:

1F.   Demonstrate willingness to trust others
1G.   Develop skills for making and maintaining relationships
1H.   Recognize and deal with peer pressure
1J.   Recognize the need for help and develop the ability to ask for it

Goal 2: Increase Self-Awareness and Self-Acceptance

Objectives:

2G.   Recognize personal boundaries, rights, and privacy needs
2H.   Identify personal and social roles

Goal 4: Increase Understanding and Valuing of Diversity

Objectives:

4A.   Recognize and appreciate individual differences
4B.   Develop an understanding and appreciation of own culture
4C.   Demonstrate respect for others as both individuals and members of different cultural groups
4D.   Acknowledge and appreciate similarities and differences across cultures and/or groups of people who have physical or learning differences

Goal 5: Demonstrate Consistently Responsible Behavior

Objectives:

5A.   Acknowledge personal responsibilities
5B.   Recognize whether behavior is appropriate and responsible
5C.   Act in an appropriate and responsible manner
5D.   Develop coping skills for dealing with stress
5E.   Understand the need for self-discipline and self-control and how to exercise them

Materials: Open space and some boundary markers (natural or artificial)

Preparation: Boundary markers if necessary

How to Play:

1.   This is a simple game of tag—with a variation of Base in which participants are safe from being tagged as It.
2.   As always, this is, for us, a WALKING game.
3.   Explain to participants that it is a game of tag (a WALKING game of tag) and that you (the leader) will begin by being It. If you tag another participant, that participant becomes It and needs to chase (by WALKING) other participants.

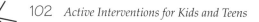

4. The important addition to a normal tag game is that participants are safe from being tagged as It only if the person is hugging one other person. Two participants hugging are safe. If more than two are hugging one another, none of them are safe.

5. In order to keep participants from simply hugging the entire game (though there might be some value in this too), clarify that the two participants can only hug as long as they can hum—on one breath. In other words, at the beginning of their hug (as they quickly come together to keep from being tagged), each participant should take a deep breath and begin to hum. They can hug as long as they can hum on that one breath. However, when they stop humming to take a breath they are no longer safe from being tagged It.

6. Once participant A has hugged participant B (for one hum), those two participants cannot hug again until they have hugged someone else. This way, participants cannot simply take a breath and hug, then take a breath and hug the same person again.

7. We recommend you (the leader) being It first. If you are It, you can move toward people and help them catch on to the value of hugging to avoid being tagged.

8. We also recommend a fairly tight space so that participants often need to hug to escape being tagged.

9. In order to slow down the transition of the person who is newly tagged to tagging others and to alert all the participants to who is It now, we like to have the newly tagged person raise his or her hands and yell, "I'm It! I'm It! I'm It!" It's also funny.

Sample Personalization-Processing Questions:

1. How did you feel about this activity? What did you like about it? What didn't you like about it? What was easy about it? What was difficult about it?

2. When you were the taggee, how did you feel when you got caught by the tagger? When you were the tagger, how did you feel when you caught the taggee? How did you feel during the transitions (changing from taggee to tagger and vice versa)?

3. Which role did you like best? What did you like about it? What did you dislike about the other role?

4. How did your level of trust of the group influence whether or not you chose to hug someone so that you would not be tagged?

5. How did your level of trust with specific people influence who you chose to hug? How did you handle it when someone you did not want to hug wanted to hug you?

6. How did peer pressure affect who you hugged?

7. What did you do when the person who was It was hot on your trail? Did you realize that you could ask for help when this was happening? How did you ask for help from others when you recognized you needed it?

8. How did you feel about having to hug someone to be safe?

9. What impact did having to hug someone to be safe have on your recognition of your personal boundaries, rights, and privacy needs?

10. Some people are comfortable hugging others, and some are not. Did you notice any differences in your willingness to hug and the willingness to hug of other people in the group?

11. What were your responsibilities to the group in this activity? How did you decide what your responsibilities were?

12. Did you honor those responsibilities in playing this activity? If yes, what kinds of things did you do that you felt were responsible? How did you make sure your behavior was responsible? If no, what kinds of things did you do that you felt were not responsible? What kept you from being responsible during this activity?

13. How could you tell whether other people perceived your behaviors as responsible? What kinds of feedback did you get from others about whether you were being responsible during this activity? How did you react when you got this kind of feedback?

14. What about this activity made it important to exercise self-discipline and self-control?

15. What did you find stressful in this activity? What strategies did you use to cope with this stress?

Sample Application-Processing Questions:

1. In other situations in your life, how comfortable are you with physical touch? How much do you have to trust someone to hug them?

2. What are some other situations in your life in which you might experience peer pressure to hug someone or allow other physical touch? How do you/will you deal with these situations?

3. What could you learn from this game that you could apply in situations in which it would be important to recognize and maintain your personal boundaries, rights, and privacy needs?
4. What are the rules (spoken or unspoken) about physical touch and/or physical closeness in your family? In your culture?
5. What are some other situations in which you have noticed differences in people's comfort levels about physical touch and/or physical closeness? What were the differences that you noticed?
6. What have you noticed about different cultural groups and their rules about physical touch and/or physical closeness?
7. If someone else has different rules than you do about physical touch and/or physical closeness, how can you handle this in an appropriate way?
8. In relationships with friends, romantic partners (depending on the age—probably don't want to include that part of the question with first and second graders, though the times they are a-changing), and family members, are you more comfortable as the pursuer or the pursued? What do you like about that role? How often do you play that role in relationships? How often do you play the other role? What is uncomfortable for you about that role?
9. Are there other roles you play in your relationships (besides pursuer or pursued)? What are they? How often do you play these roles? How comfortable are you in each of these roles?
10. What are some situations or relationships in which you feel that it is really important to act in a responsible manner? How do you handle these situations or relationships?
11. What are some times when you do not act as responsibly as you think you should? What do you think keeps you from being more responsible in those situations? How could you handle those situations differently in the future?
12. How do you feel when you get feedback that you are not acting in a responsible manner? How do you react to this feedback? How is your reaction affected by who it is that is giving the feedback? The way the feedback is delivered?
13. How do you handle situations in which friends or family members are not acting responsibly? What kinds of feedback do you usually give in these situations? How do you handle situations in which acquaintances or strangers are not acting responsibly? What kinds of feedback do you usually give in these situations?
14. In what kinds of situations in your life do you feel the same kind of stress you felt during this activity? How can you apply what you learned in this activity about how you handle stress to those other situations?
15. What are some other situations in your life in which it is important to exercise self-control and self-discipline? How can you apply what you learned during this activity about your ability to exercise self-control and self-discipline to these situations?
16. What are some other situations in your life in which a person's willingness to act in a responsible manner can affect your ability to trust him or her?

Safety Concerns: None, as long as folks are WALKING—

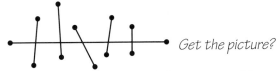
Get the picture?

Name of Activity: Human Camera

Type of Activity: Trust

Grade Level: Seventh grade and up

Size of Group: 2 to 16

Goal 2: Increase Self-Awareness and Self-Acceptance

Objectives:

2A.   Explore personal attitudes and values
2B.   Identify and acknowledge personal positive traits, talents, and accomplishments
2E.   Appreciate own uniqueness
2F.   Develop positive attitudes toward self
2G.   Recognize personal boundaries, rights, and privacy needs

Goal 4: Increase Understanding and Valuing of Diversity

Objectives:

4A.   Recognize and appreciate individual differences
4B.   Develop an understanding and appreciation of own culture
4C.   Demonstrate respect for others as both individuals and members of different cultural groups
4D.   Acknowledge and appreciate similarities and differences across cultures and/or groups of people who have physical or learning differences
4E.   Recognize how stereotypes can affect interpersonal relationships and attitudes toward others

Goal 5: Demonstrate Consistently Responsible Behavior

Objectives:

5A.   Acknowledge personal responsibilities
5B.   Recognize whether behavior is appropriate and responsible
5C.   Act in an appropriate and responsible manner
5E.   Understand the need for self-discipline and self-control and how to exercise them
5G.   Demonstrate respect for alternate perspectives

Materials: None

Preparation: None

How to Play:

1.   Have the group pair up.
2.   Within each pair, designate one person to be the photographer and one person to be the camera.
3.   While the camera keeps his or her eyes closed, the photographer physically guides the camera (e.g., hands on shoulders) on a search for interesting photographs. When the photographer finds an interesting photograph, he or she positions the camera and frames the object by moving the head into position for the eyes to view the image and then presses the shutter button (by tapping on the camera's shoulder). After a 3- to 5-second exposure time, photographers should close the shutter button (by tapping on the camera's shoulder). The 3- to 5-second exposure time is perfect to imprint the image in the camera's mind. With longer exposures, the camera's mind begins to wander, reducing the impact of the photograph. Be sure to encourage cameras to keep their eyes shut between pictures to heighten the impact of the photograph.

4. Photographers can prepare their cameras for the next picture by telling them what kind of lens to use (i.e., telescopic, wide angle, movie—in which the photographer slowly moves the camera).
5. Have the photographers take four to six pictures (or give them a 5- to 10-minute time frame) and then return to the starting place where roles can be reversed.
6. This activity can be played anywhere. Be sure to encourage the photographers to be creative in what they photograph.[1]

Variations:

1. This activity can be used in a variety of different ways. For example, participants can be told to take pictures with their human camera that demonstrate diversity (or lack of diversity) present in their school. Following this activity, discussion could center on what diversity is and how we create a more diverse school/neighborhood.
2. This activity can also be used as a closing activity after a semester or term of working in a specific group.
3. Other possibilities for this activity:
   a. Encourage the photographers to create a photo essay connected to a specific theme (e.g., nature appreciation, trust).
   b. Have photographers create a memory album of the memories of a specific day or class.
   c. Have photographers give their camera a gift by way of a photograph.
   d. Have all the participants be cameras at the same time. Have them hold onto a rope and pull them along gently to the next picture with their eyes closed. This technique could be used in preparing a group for a number of different initiatives. As an orientation, you could take photographs of the various activities that you are going to do throughout your time together.
   e. Use a visualization. If photographers cannot find the right picture, have them lie down in a grassy area and describe the picture to the camera (who still has his or her eyes closed).
4. After each person has played both roles, give all the group members a 3- by 5-inch card and tell them to remember one of the pictures they took when they played the camera. Develop it by drawing it on the card and giving it back to the photographer.
5. Have participants close their eyes and think back to the activity or activities they have recently completed. Within these activities, have them visualize themselves at their best, a moment when they surpassed their own expectations. Tell participants to remember this picture of themselves in the future when they need strength to complete a difficult task.
6. If possible, you may want to try to take an actual photograph of each participant in the group doing something right. These pictures could be given to participants at the end of the group as a reminder of the group experience.
7. To frame this activity, you can, for example, bring in a photograph and discuss why it is important for us to develop memories. What do memories tell us about ourselves? Stress the importance of making positive memories in which we visualize ourselves as successful. Discuss how we can help one another make positive memories in our classroom or group.

Sample Personalization-Processing Questions:

1. When you were the photographer, how did you decide what to photograph? How did you decide which kind of lens to use?
2. How did what you chose to photograph reflect your personal attitudes and values? How did it reflect your uniqueness?
3. When you were the camera, what did you think/feel about the scenes your photographer chose? How did you express your thoughts/feelings?
4. Did you feel free to give constructive feedback to your photographer? What determined whether you felt free to give constructive feedback to your photographer?
5. Which role did you like best? What did you like about the role you preferred? What did you dislike about the role you liked least?
6. When you were the camera, how did it feel to have the photographer position your head or touch your shoulders? Were there any issues connected to your personal boundaries, rights, and privacy needs when this happened?

_____
[1]*Note.* Adapted from Cornell, J. (1989). *Sharing the joy of nature.* Nevada City, CA: Dawn.

7. How did you feel about wandering around with your eyes closed?
8. When you were the photographer, how did you make sure that you did not touch your partner in a way that was uncomfortable to him or her? If your partner did touch you in a way that was uncomfortable for you, how did you give feedback to him or her?
9. When you were the camera, did you keep your eyes closed the entire time you were supposed to? How did your level of trust of your partner influence whether or not you chose to keep your eyes closed?
10. When you were the camera, what method did you use to help you remember the scene you were supposed to be photographing? If you had trouble remembering the scene you were supposed to be photographing, how did you feel about this?
11. How did you feel about someone else controlling your movement?
12. How did your family values and attitudes affect what you chose to photograph? How did your cultural values and attitudes affect what you chose to photograph?
13. How were the scenes you chose to photograph different from the scenes that your partner chose to photograph? How were the scenes you chose to photograph different from the scenes that others in the group chose to photograph?
14. Did you notice any patterns across the members in the group related to the scenes people chose to photograph? What were those patterns? Were those patterns related in any way to the culture of those taking the photographs?
15. Did you notice any stereotypes you were holding about certain people in this process? How did your holding those stereotypes affect how you interpreted what they chose to photograph?
16. What were your responsibilities to your partner in this activity? How did you decide what your responsibilities were?
17. Did you honor those responsibilities to your partner? If yes, what kinds of things did you do that you felt were responsible? How did you make sure your behavior was responsible? If no, what kinds of things did you do that you felt were not responsible? What kept you from being more responsible during this activity?
18. How could you tell whether your partner perceived your behaviors as responsible? What kinds of feedback did you get from your partner about whether you were being responsible during this activity? How did you react when you got this kind of feedback?
19. What about this activity made it important to exercise self-discipline and self-control?

Sample Application-Processing Questions:

1. In other situations in your life, how comfortable are you with physical touch? How much do you have to trust someone to touch them? Allow them to touch you?
2. What are some other situations in your life in which you feel as if you are going into something blindly? How do you feel about those situations? How do you handle those situations?
3. How do you usually decide whether to trust or not trust? How are your behaviors and reactions different in situations in which you are trusting versus situations in which you are not trusting?
4. What could you learn from this activity that you could apply in situations in which it would be important to recognize and maintain your personal boundaries, rights, and privacy needs?
5. What are the rules (spoken or unspoken) about physical touch and/or physical closeness in your family? In your culture?
6. What are some other situations in which you have noticed differences in people's comfort levels about physical touch and/or physical closeness? What were the differences that you noticed? If someone else has different rules than you do about physical touch and/or physical closeness, how can you handle this in an appropriate, respectful way?
7. What have you noticed about different cultural groups and their rules about physical touch and/or physical closeness?
8. What are some situations or relationships when you feel that it is really important to act in a responsible manner? How do you handle these situations or relationships?
9. What are some times when you do not act as responsibly as you think you should? What do you think keeps you from being more responsible in those situations? How could you handle those situations differently in the future?

10. How do you feel when you get feedback that you are not acting in a responsible manner? How do you react to this feedback? How is your reaction affected by who it is that is giving the feedback? By the way the feedback is delivered?

11. What are some other situations in your life in which it is important to exercise self-control and self-discipline? How can you apply what you learned during this activity about your ability to exercise self-control and self-discipline to these situations?

12. What are some other situations in your life in which a person's willingness to act in a responsible manner can affect your ability to trust him or her?

13. What are some other situations in your life in which you could notice and celebrate your own uniqueness? Your successes?

14. How do you usually handle situations in which your perspective differs from that of others? What is it important to communicate in those situations? How can you communicate about your perspective in a way that maximizes the chances that you will be heard, understood, and respected?

Safety Concerns: Make sure folks don't wander off blindly, hit walls, or trip over obstacles. This is why you have those herders to help you if the crowd is large.

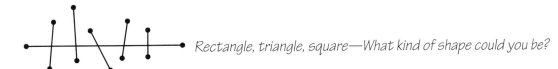

Rectangle, triangle, square—What kind of shape could you be?

Name of Activity: Human Shapes

Type of Activity: *Trust; Challenge/Initiative*

Grade Level: *Third grade and up*

Size of Group: *8 to 24*

Goal 1: Improve Communication and Relationship Skills

Objectives:

1D.   Express ideas clearly and constructively
1E.   Listen actively to others
1I.   Use communication skills to resolve conflict
1J.   Recognize the need for help and develop the ability to ask for it
1K.   Recognize and verbalize needs and wishes
1L.   Develop skills for effectively participating in groups

Goal 3: Develop and Apply Problem-Solving and Decision-Making Skills

Objectives:

3B.   Identify problems
3C.   Demonstrate understanding of steps for solving problems and making decisions (gather information; explore alternatives and consequences; plan and take action)
3D.   Evaluate decisions
3H.   Demonstrate effective coping skills for dealing with problems
3I.   Recognize when peer pressure is influencing decision making
3J.   Develop ability to identify alternative methods for solving problems and achieving goals

Goal 5: Demonstrate Consistently Responsible Behavior

Objectives:

5D.   Develop coping skills for dealing with stress
5G.   Demonstrate respect for alternate perspectives

Goal 6: Enhance Positive Attitudes and Skills Related to Learning

Objectives:

6A.   Develop feeling of competence and confidence as a learner
6B.   Take pride in accomplishments
6C.   Accept mistakes as part of the learning process
6E.   Recognize that effort and persistence enhance learning
6G.   Develop the ability to share knowledge
6H.   Develop critical-thinking skills

Materials:

1.   One piece of rope or tubular webbing long enough to account for roughly 6 feet of rope per participant
2.   One blindfold for each participant—unless you will have them simply close their eyes (which has pros and cons)

Preparation: None

How to Play:

1. In this activity participants make different shapes out of the rope or webbing they are holding on to. The trick is to do this without the use of your sight. No peeking—but talking is okay and might actually be necessary.
2. Begin by blindfolding everyone in the group (or have them close their eyes).
3. Have participants spread out roughly equally distant from each other and hold on to the rope, webbing, string, or whatever you are using (with at least one hand).
4. Instruct the group that, without removing their blindfolds or letting go of the rope, they should arrange themselves so that the rope forms a specific geometric figure—square, circle, triangle, hexagon, go wild!
5. After the participants in the group think they are done, invite them to take off their blindfolds or open their eyes to see how they did.
6. Sometimes we encourage the group to plan a strategy before they try the next shape.

Variations:

1. Sometimes we divide the group into subgroups, each with their own piece of rope, etc. It can be a competition (e.g., which group makes the best triangle?) or a collaborative effort (e.g., two groups each making a triangle with the points touching so that together they look a little like a bowtie).
2. Sometimes we alternate having participants be able to (a) talk and see (not blindfolded), (b) talk but be blindfolded, and (c) not talk and be blindfolded, and have them talk about the difference. It is really interesting to note that people prefer different ways.

Sample Personalization-Processing Questions:

1. What did you feel/think about the group's chances for success when the leader first explained the rules? How did you express your thoughts and feelings to the other members of the group?
2. How successful was your group with this activity? How did you define success? Did the different members of your group define success differently? How did these differences affect the communication and cooperation in the group?
3. If your group failed, how was that for you? How did you handle this failure? What did you tell yourself about yourself and your abilities related to this failure? What did you tell yourself about other members of your group related to this failure? How could you have dealt with this more constructively?
4. If your group was successful, how was that for you? How did you handle this success? What did you tell yourself about yourself and your abilities related to this success? What did you tell yourself about other members of your group related to this success?
5. If there were a number of small groups doing this activity, did you compare your group to other groups? What effect did this comparison have on you? Did you compare yourself to the other members of your group? What effect did this comparison have on you?
6. How important was communication between you and the other members of your group in this activity?
7. Did you feel heard by the other members of your group as you worked on making the shapes? Did you feel heard by the other members of your group if you stopped to strategize? If you did feel heard, how was that for you? If you didn't feel heard, how was that for you?
8. If you only felt heard some of the time, what do you think determined whether you were heard? If you had wanted to be heard more consistently by the other members of the group, what could you have done differently to make sure that you were heard?
9. Did you communicate your ideas effectively? Did you communicate your needs and wishes effectively? If so, how did you go about doing this? If not, what prevented you from doing this? How could you go about communicating your ideas, needs, and wishes more effectively?
10. Why was listening important in this activity? How did you do as a listener in this activity? How could you have improved your listening?
11. What role did trust play in this activity? What could you and the other members of the group have done to enhance trust in the group?
12. What process did the members of the group use to determine how to go about making the shapes? How did the members of the group decide whether a strategy was working? If a strategy wasn't working, how did the group deal with that? How did you go about developing an alternative strategy when something wasn't working?

13. If you were making shapes that didn't really look like the shape you wanted to make, how did you apply what you learned from these mistakes to perfect what the group was doing?

14. Why was cooperation important in this activity? What were some of the ways that the members of the group cooperated with one another to accomplish this task? How did cooperation help?

15. How did you decide whether to cooperate or not? How did your attitudes about cooperation influence what happened among the members of the group?

16. How could you tell whether you needed more help from the other members of the group? What did you do when you needed more help? How did you ask for more help when you recognized you needed it?

17. What role did you play in this process (leader? follower? observer?)? Did the group need someone to be the leader to be able to make the shapes? If so, how did you work out who was going to lead and who was going to follow? Did the roles change during the course of the activity? How?

18. If group members disagreed on strategies for making the shapes, did you define that disagreement as conflict? If yes, how did you feel about the conflict? What did you do about your feelings? How did the members of the group resolve the conflict? What would have been some other ways to do this?

19. How did you feel about it when the group was successful at making a shape?

20. How did you react when other people had ideas different from yours about how to make the shapes? How did you decide which ideas were ideas the group should try?

21. If you did the variation in which sometimes you are blind (-folded) and sometimes not, sometimes you can talk and other times you can't, which combination worked best for your group? What was the advantage of being blindfolded but able to talk? What was the advantage of being able to see but not able to talk? What was the advantage of being able to see and to talk?

22. On a 1 to 10 scale, how stressful was this activity for you? What made it stressful? Where did you feel the stress in your body? What could have been done to make the activity less stressful for you?

23. Were there any instances in which peer pressure affected the group members during this process? What impact did peer pressure have on you? What did you do to cope with peer pressure?

Sample Application-Processing Questions:

1. In what other situations or relationships in your life does it feels as though you must work with other people to make something happen? What resources/strategies do you have to help you deal with these situations?

2. What part does cooperation play in these situations or relationships? How do you elicit cooperation and help?

3. In other situations in your life, how do you decide what role you are going to play?

4. In what other situations or relationships in your life does it feel as though you are trying to do something without being able to see what is going on? How do these situations affect you? How do you feel in these situations? What strategies do you use to cope with these situations? How can you apply what you learned in this activity to these situations?

5. In what other situations or relationships in your life does it feel as though you can't communicate with others about what is happening? How do these situations affect you? How do you feel in these situations? What strategies do you use to cope with these situations? How can you apply what you learned in this activity to these situations?

6. How do you usually go about solving problems? Which of the methods for problem solving used by the members of the group would be useful in other situations in your life? How can you use them in these situations?

7. What are some other situations in which you might need to ask for help? How can you go about recognizing that you need help and asking for it?

8. What are some other situations or relationships in which it might be important for you to be heard? How can you go about making sure that you are heard in those situations?

9. What are some other situations or relationships in which it might be important for you to be a good listener? How can you go about making sure that you are using effective listening skills in those situations?

10. What are some other situations or relationships in which you need to use your conflict resolution skills? How can you apply some of the methods that you learned/practiced in this activity for appropriately resolving conflicts in these situations?

11. What could you learn from this activity that you could apply in situations in which it would be important to share information with others? Use critical-thinking skills?

12. What are some other situations in your life in which trusting others is important? How can you apply what you learned about trusting others in this activity to those other situations?

13. What are some other situations in which you have felt as if you had failed? How have you handled these situations? How can you apply what you learned in this activity to those situations?

14. What are some other situations or relationships in which you compare yourself to others? What has the impact of those comparisons been on you and/or your relationships? How can you apply what you learned in this activity about comparing yourself to others to those situations or relationships?

15. In what kind of situation in your life do you decide to be a leader? How do you go about leading? In what kind of situation in your life do you decide to be a follower? How do you go about following? In what kind of situation in your life do you decide to be an observer? How do you go about observing?

Safety Concerns: None

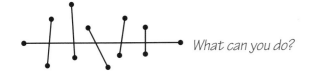 *What can you do?*

Name of Activity: I Can Do This!!

Type of Activity: Icebreaker; Deinhibitizer

Grade Level: First grade and up

Size of Group: 2 to 20—many more takes more time

Goal 2: Increase Self-Awareness and Self-Acceptance

Objectives:

2B.   Identify and acknowledge personal positive traits, talents, and accomplishments
2E.   Appreciate own uniqueness

Goal 4: Increase Understanding and Valuing of Diversity

Objectives:

4A.   Recognize and appreciate individual differences
4C.   Demonstrate respect for others as both individuals and members of different cultural groups
4E.   Recognize how stereotypes can affect interpersonal relationships and attitudes toward others

Materials: None

Preparation: None

How to Play:

1.   In this activity each member of the group shows what he or she can do, and everybody tries it!
2.   Have the group form a circle with enough room for some movement and in which all the participants can see each other.
3.   We like to explain to groups that we all have lots of talents and abilities, some rare and unique, some that others share. This activity is about discovering and trying those things out.
4.   Each participant around the circle shows a specific thing that he or she can do and then the entire group tries it.
5.   We usually go first by showing the group what we can do. For instance, Jeff can jump up and kick his heels—though we try to restrain him from breaking into song ("Oklahoma! Where the wind comes rushing down the plain!"—not pretty). Don can bend his index finger at only the first joint without bending the second one—pretty tricky.
6.   Do note that by going first you model that the thing you are showing is physical (can be seen and thus imitated by others) and isn't necessarily dramatic (unless you fall over trying to kick your heels).
7.   A round of applause follows each person's illustration of what he or she can do.
8.   We usually go around the circle showing what we can do. However, we do allow participants to pass so they can think of something. We just come back to them at the end. We also make it clear that you can do the same thing that someone else has done (so no one will necessarily take your thing).
9.   Finally, we usually have a couple of ideas in our head that we're pretty sure a person could do and are happy to suggest it in a stage whisper if some seems stuck.

Sample Personalization-Processing Questions:

1.   How did you decide what you wanted to show the group as your talent or ability?
2.   How did it feel when everybody else in the group tried to duplicate your talent or ability? What was your reaction when others were successful in duplicating your talent or ability? What was your reaction when others were unsuccessful in duplicating your talent or ability?

3. How did it feel when the other members of the group acknowledged your talent or ability?
4. Were there patterns in the talents or activities that group members chose to demonstrate? What did you notice about those patterns?
5. Were there any talents or activities that surprised you?
6. How did you demonstrate respect for the talents and activities of others in the group?
7. Did you notice any stereotypes you were holding about certain people in this process? How did your holding those stereotypes affect how you interacted with those people?
8. If you chose to pass and never demonstrated a talent or activity, how do you feel about that? Do you wish you had made a different choice? Would you like to demonstrate a talent or activity now?

Sample Application-Processing Questions:

1. What are some other situations in which you demonstrate your talents or abilities to other people? How do you feel about those situations?
2. What are other situations in which you get to teach others talents or activities you know how to do? How do you feel about these experiences?
3. What are other situations in which others acknowledge your talents or activities? How do you feel about these experiences?
4. What did you learn about yourself in this process? How can you apply what you learned about yourself in other situations in your life?
5. How can you enhance your awareness of the talents and activities of others in your life? How can you more consistently demonstrate respect for these talents and activities?
6. How can stereotypes affect your interpersonal relationships and attitudes toward others? What are some things you can do to prevent this from happening?
7. Are there other situations or relationships in your life in which you avoid participating in experiences and/or demonstrating your talents and accomplishments? How do you feel about this avoidance? What, if anything, would you like to do to change this pattern?
8. How can you learn to more fully appreciate your own uniqueness?

Safety Concerns: None

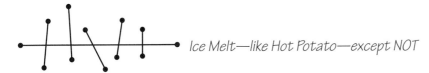 *Ice Melt—like Hot Potato—except NOT*

Name of Activity: Ice Melt

Type of Activity: *Icebreaker*

Grade Level: *Third grade and up*

Size of Group: *8 to 16*

Goal 1: Improve Communication and Relationship Skills

Objectives:

  1D.   Express ideas clearly and constructively
  1H.   Recognize and deal with peer pressure
  1L.   Develop skills for effectively participating in groups

Goal 2: Increase Self-Awareness and Self-Acceptance

Objectives:

  2A.   Explore personal attitudes and values
  2B.   Identify and acknowledge personal positive traits, talents, and accomplishments
  2E.   Appreciate own uniqueness
  2F.   Develop positive attitudes toward self
  2H.   Identify personal and social roles

Goal 4: Increase Understanding and Valuing of Diversity

Objectives:

  4A.   Recognize and appreciate individual differences
  4B.   Develop an understanding and appreciation of own culture
  4C.   Demonstrate respect for others as both individuals and members of different cultural groups
  4D.   Acknowledge and appreciate similarities and differences across cultures and/or groups of people who have physical or learning differences

Materials: Ice cubes or crushed ice

Preparation: None

How to Play:

1.   Have the group form a circle with all participants facing inward.
2.   Have one participant (or you, if you'd like to model how the game is played) take a handful of ice cubes or crushed ice. We often place the ice in a plastic bag so that there is less dripping as the ice melts. A nice big bag of ice held in two hands is perfect (unless you're the one holding it—it's cold!).
3.   The participant with the ice stands directly in front of one of the people standing in the circle.
4.   The participant who the leader (i.e., ice holder) has chosen to stand in front of must simply talk about him- or herself.
5.   However, when the person talking (who has the ice holder in front of him or her) pauses (this includes taking an extra long breath or saying "um"), the ice gets passed to that person, and he or she holds the ice and finds someone new to stand in front of (while the now previous ice holder takes that person's place in the circle).
6.   Note that *any* pause at all is not allowed, and the individuals in the group serve as judges of this by raising one hand when they believe a pause has occurred. Once the majority of hands are in the air, the two people (i.e., the ice holder and the person who was talking) must trade places.

Variations:

Ask participants to focus on their cultural heritage as they talk.

Sample Personalization-Processing Questions:

1. How did it feel to be the center of attention, talking about yourself?
2. How did you decide what to tell the group about yourself? What kinds of things did you say (positive things, negative things, accomplishments, mistakes, funny things, etc.)?
3. How were the things you talked about different from the things that others told? What did you notice about your uniqueness?
4. How were the things you told about yourself similar to the things that other people told about themselves? What did you notice about having in common with others in the group?
5. How did what you discussed express your personal attitudes and values?
6. How did you feel when the person with the ice decided to stand in front of you—making you the next person to talk? As that person talked, how did you prepare to be the next person who was going to talk?
7. How did you feel about having to give the ice to someone else? How did you decide who was going to be the next person to get the ice/talk? How did peer pressure affect who you gave the ice to? How did you deal with that peer pressure?
8. What were some of the roles you play that you mentioned when you talked? How do you feel about those roles?
9. How did you deal with it if the other members of the group thought you had paused when you did not believe that you had?
10. How did your culture influence how you felt about talking? How did your culture influence what you said?
11. What did you notice about other people's cultures as they talked?

Sample Application-Processing Questions:

1. What are some other situations in which you are the center of attention? How do you feel about those situations? How do you handle those situations?
2. When you have to talk in front of a group, how do you decide what to say? What impact does the setting have on what you decide to say?
3. What are some of your personal positive traits, talents, and accomplishments? Where do you get to celebrate those positive qualities?
4. What are some ways you are unique? What are some other situations in which you notice your own uniqueness? How can you celebrate that uniqueness?
5. What are some other situations in which you notice you have things in common with others? What kind of things do you have in common with others in those situations?
6. What are some other situations in which you might have to deal with peer pressure? How do you usually handle those situations? How can you apply what you might have learned about handling peer pressure in this activity to those situations?
7. How can you apply what you learned about handling situations in which you disagree with the other members of a group to other relationships in your life?
8. What are some of the roles you usually play in your relationships? What impact will what you learned about roles in this activity have on those relationships?
9. What ways does your culture influence your actions and relationships? How can you become more aware of how your culture affects your actions and relationships? How can you become more aware of how other people's cultures affect their actions and relationships?
10. How can you apply what you have learned today about your own culture and the cultures of others to reduce the number of stereotypes you hold and help you view other people in a more realistic and respectful way?
11. How do your personal attitudes and values have an impact on your relationships? How can what you learned in this activity about your personal attitudes and values help you in expressing your values and attitudes in constructive ways?

Safety Concerns: None apart from the possible wet floor from the melting ice.

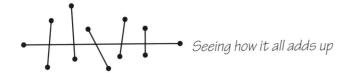
Seeing how it all adds up

Name of Activity: Keypunch

Type of Activity: Challenge/Initiative

Grade Level: Fourth grade and up

Size of Group: 4 to 20

Goal 1: Improve Communication and Relationship Skills

Objectives:

1B. Express feelings clearly and constructively
1C. Recognize and accept the feelings of others
1D. Express ideas clearly and constructively
1E. Listen actively to others
1H. Recognize and deal with peer pressure
1I. Use communications skills to resolve conflict
1J. Recognize the need for help and develop the ability to ask for it
1L. Develop skills for effectively participating in groups

Goal 2: Increase Self-Awareness and Self-Acceptance

Objectives:

2B. Identify and acknowledge personal positive traits, talents, and accomplishments
2C. Develop ability to recognize negative self-talk
2D. Develop skills in replacing negative self-talk with positive self-talk
2F. Develop positive attitudes toward self
2H. Identify personal and social roles

Goal 3: Develop and Apply Problem-Solving and Decision-Making Skills

Objectives:

3A. Set personal goals
3B. Identify problems
3C. Demonstrate understanding of steps for solving problems and making decisions (gather information; explore alternatives and consequences; plan and take action)
3D. Evaluate decisions
3F. Apply decision-making skills to resolve conflicts
3G. Apply decision-making skills in life situations
3H. Demonstrate effective coping skills for dealing with problems
3I. Recognize when peer pressure is influencing decision making
3J. Develop ability to identify alternative methods for solving problems and achieving goals

Goal 5: Demonstrate Consistently Responsible Behavior

Objectives:

5A. Acknowledge personal responsibilities
5B. Recognize whether behavior is appropriate and responsible
5C. Act in an appropriate and responsible manner
5D. Develop coping skills for dealing with stress
5E. Understand the need for self-discipline and self-control and how to exercise them
5G. Demonstrate respect for alternate perspectives

Goal 6: Enhance Positive Attitudes and Skills Related to Learning

Objectives:

6A. Develop feeling of competence and confidence as a learner
6B. Take pride in accomplishments
6C. Accept mistakes as part of the learning process
6D. Apply time management and task management strategies
6E. Recognize that effort and persistence enhance learning
6G. Develop the ability to share knowledge
6H. Develop critical-thinking skills

Materials: A boundary marker (e.g., rope, string, yarn, tape, or—if you're outside—chalk) and 30 plastic lids or other place markers (again, chalk if you're outside). You'll also need a digital watch with a seconds option or a watch or clock with a second hand so you can time the group.

Preparation: Write the numbers 1 to 30 on the 30 plastic lids and place the lids, number side up, in a random array inside the circular boundary. Note that it doesn't have to be a circle, we just tend to think that way, and that the diameter of the closed, geometric-shaped boundary (or circle for the rest of us) can be from 8 to 15 feet depending on how spread out you'd like the numbers, and how much room you have. If you're using chalk, simply draw a big circle with 30 smaller circles inside it with the numbers 1 to 30 written in random order inside those smaller circles.

How to Play:

1. We like to explain the game to participants a few feet (or outside, a few yards) away from the circle.
2. When you are standing nearby—but not too close to the boundary—explain to the group that the goal is for the group to touch the numbers from 1 to 30 in consecutive order (1, then 2, then 3) as quickly as possible, and that you will be timing them. We typically don't clarify HOW the participants have to touch each number (e.g., with a hand, foot, nose), just that they have to physically touch it.
3. Explain that there are several rules that must be followed:
   - First: Only one member of the group needs to touch a number (e.g., if Billy touches number 1 that counts as the group touching it; all the group members do not need to touch each number; someone from the group must touch each number).
   - Second: No person can touch two consecutive numbers (e.g., if Billy touches number 1, he cannot touch number 2. After somebody else touches number 2, Billy could touch number 3, but if he does, he cannot touch number 4).
   - Third: Only one person is allowed inside the boundary perimeter at a time (e.g., if Billy touches number 1, Suzie cannot jump in and touch number 2 until Billy is outside of the circle).
   - Fourth: All members of the group must participate.
   - Fifth: This is a WALKING activity (sometimes we practice walking just to reinforce this).
   - Sixth: There are TIME penalties for breaking all of the preceding rules including touching numbers out of sequence (1, 2, 4, oops).
   - Seventh: Finally explain that the group will get three (or two or seven depending on your preference and how much time you have) attempts to complete the task as quickly as possible and that they are going for a world record!
4. Depending on your group, set the time penalties at 10, 15, 20, or 30 seconds. You will keep track of the group's time (from when they leave your designated starting area, where you explained the activity, to when they complete the activity and return to that area) and add the penalties (5 penalties at 10 seconds a penalty would be 50 seconds added to their time).
5. Depending on your group, give them some time to plan, and then get them started on their first try. We like to explain the rules over and over (so you may want to write them on a note card—we do because our memories are so bad).
6. During the group's tries at the activity, watch for penalties. Note particularly whether there is more than one person in the circle at a time. Also watch for touching numbers out of sequence. Early on participants will inadvertently touch other numbers as they try to move across the circle to a specific number. When you later explain this penalty to them, a light bulb often goes on for them.

7. There is lots to watch for in this activity! The hard part is trying to figure out who will touch which number, and if we both think we should touch a number then we both enter the circle at the same time—oops! There's another penalty.
8. At the end of the activity we like to congratulate the group on how well they did and let them know that, in fact, they set a world record. We like to say, "That was absolutely the fastest we have ever seen you do that—" which usually gets a groan.

Variations:

There are a seemingly infinite number of variations of Keypunch. Some of our favorites include

1. Doing the activity as a three-legged race. That is, every participant has his or her ankle tied to that of another participant. Takes some cooperation and is silly!
2. Making the rule that only one participant can be breaking the plane of the circle. In that way, anybody who points at a number (Ooh! Ooh! There's 17!) and has his or her arm extended over the plane of the boundary gets a penalty!
3. Making the rule that only two feet can be touching inside the circle at time. Sometimes participants choose to try to hop! Sometimes they figure out that they can lean way into the circle on hands and knees, as long as they keep their feet outside.
4. Making the rule that you have to touch the numbers with your hand.
5. Adding the rule that during the planning time the group can talk all they want, but when the activity starts there is no talking, and there is a penalty for each violation as for any other rule.
6. Sometimes we give the group a couple of tries, and then change the rules to some of those just listed here noting whether/how the group's time changes.

Sample Personalization-Processing Questions:

1. What did you feel/think about the group's chances for success when the leader first explained the rules? How did you express your thoughts and feelings? How did your initial attitude affect your approach to solving the problem?
2. What did you do to contribute to the group touching the numbers in the correct order? What did you do to contribute to the group doing the activity as quickly as possible? How did you feel about your contribution?
3. If your group didn't successfully complete the activity or took too long to do it, how was that for you? How did you handle this failure? What did you tell yourself about yourself and your abilities related to this failure? What did you tell yourself about the other group members' abilities related to this failure? How could you have dealt with this more constructively?
4. If your group successfully beat the world's record, how was that for you? How did you handle this success? What did you tell yourself about yourself and your abilities related to this success? What did you tell yourself about the other group members and their abilities related to this success? Was there some way you could have dealt with this more constructively?
5. If the group did the activity successfully and the leader challenged you to beat your own time, how did you feel about this? If the group did the activity successfully and the leader changed the rules, how did you feel about this?
6. How important was communication between you and the other members of the group in this activity? What did you do to make sure that the communication among group members was appropriate, clear, and constructive?
7. Did you feel heard by the other members of the group as you developed a strategy to complete the activity? How did it feel when you were heard by the other group members?
8. If you didn't feel heard, what was that like for you? If you had wanted to be heard by the other members of the group, what could you have done differently to make sure that you were heard?
9. Did you communicate your ideas and feelings effectively? If so, how did you go about doing this? If not, what prevented you from doing this?
10. How did you do as a listener in this activity? How could you have improved your listening?
11. What process did you and the other members of the group use to determine how to go about completing the activity? How did you decide whether a strategy was working? If a strategy wasn't working, how did you deal with that? How did you go about developing an alternative strategy when something wasn't working?

12. What were some of the ways that members of the group cooperated with one another to accomplish this task? How did cooperation help?
13. How could you tell whether you needed more help from the other members of the group? What did you do when you needed more help? How did you ask for more help when you recognized you needed it?
14. What roles did each member of the group play in the process of completing the activity? Did one of you need to be the leader to have the group be successful? If so, how did you work out who was going to lead and who was going to follow? Did the roles change during the course of the activity? How?
15. If you and the other members of the group disagreed on strategies for completing the activity, how did you feel about the disagreement? What did you do about your feelings? Did the disagreement escalate into a conflict? How did you deal with the conflict? What would have been some other ways to do this?
16. What happened in the group if someone messed up and the group got a time penalty? Did the reaction of the group members change as time passed and things got more tense?
17. If the person who messed up was you, how did you feel? How did you handle it if this happened? How did the rest of the group react to you? How do you wish the group had reacted?
18. If the person who messed up was someone else, how did you feel? How did you handle it when this happened? How do you wish you had reacted? How did the rest of the group react to the person who messed up? How do you wish the group had reacted?
19. If you were feeling discouraged and/or frustrated in this process, how did you deal with that? What did you tell yourself to motivate yourself to continue? If other members of the group were feeling discouraged, how did you interact with them about the discouragement?
20. What did you (or the other members of the group) learn from failed attempts to complete the activity in timely fashion? How did you use that learning to perfect your strategies for perfecting your technique?
21. What were your responsibilities to the group in this activity? How did you decide what your responsibilities were?
22. Did you honor those responsibilities in doing this activity? If yes, what kinds of things did you do that you felt were responsible? How did you make sure your behavior was responsible? If no, what kinds of things did you do that you felt were not responsible? What kept you from being more responsible?
23. Were there times when you were telling yourself negative things about the group's ability to complete the activity in a timely fashion? Were there times when you were telling yourself negative things about your ability to make a positive contribution to the group completing the activity in a timely fashion? What kinds of things were you telling yourself?
24. How could you have changed this negative self-talk to more positive self-talk? What kinds of positive things could you tell yourself?
25. What part did effort and persistence play in whether you and the other members of the group were successful in completing the activity in a timely manner?
26. As you were working on completing the activity, did you compare your contribution to the process to the contribution of others? How did that comparison affect you and your efforts?
27. Why was acting with self-discipline and self-control important in this activity?
28. How was it for you to not be in control of the situation—to have to depend on others for success? How did you handle your reaction? How do you wish you had reacted?
29. How stressful was this activity for you? What made it stressful? What were some things you could you have done to make it less stressful? If you did those things, hip hip hooray! If you didn't, what kept you from doing them?

Sample Application-Processing Questions:

1. In what other situations or relationships in your life does it feel as though you must work with other people to make something happen? What resources/strategies do you have to help you deal with these situations?
2. What part does cooperation play in these situations or relationships? How do you elicit cooperation and help?

3. How did the role you had in the group resemble your role in your family? With friends? How flexible are you about roles?
4. How do you go about solving problems that are similar to the situation in this activity? Which of the methods for problem solving used by you and the members of the group would be useful in other situations in your life? How can you use them in those situations?
5. What are some other situations in which you might need to ask for help? How can you go about recognizing that you need help and asking for it? What are some other situations in which you might need to ask for what you want and/or need? How can you go about recognizing that you want and/or need something and asking for it?
6. What are some other situations or relationships in which it might be important for you to be heard? How can you go about making sure that you are heard in those situations?
7. What are some other situations or relationships in which it might be important for you to be a good listener? How can you go about making sure that you are using effective listening skills in those situations?
8. How can you apply some of the methods for communicating about feelings and ideas, encouraging cooperation, solving problems, and/or appropriately resolving conflicts that you learned/practiced in this activity in other situations?
9. How can you apply what you learned about dealing with negative self-talk?
10. What could you learn from this game that you could apply in situations in which it would be important to share information with others?
11. What did you learn about your critical-thinking skills that you can apply to other situations in your life?
12. What are some other situations in your life in which taking responsibility is important? How can you apply what you learned in this activity about taking responsibility to those other situations?
13. What are some other situations in your life in which trusting others is important? How can you apply what you learned in this activity about trusting others to those other situations?
14. What are some other situations in which you have felt like a success? How have you handled these situations? How can you apply what you learned in this activity to those situations?
15. What are some other situations in which you have felt like a failure? How have you handled these situations? How can you apply what you learned in this activity to those situations?
16. What are some other situations or relationships in which you compare yourself to others? What has the impact of those comparisons been on you and/or your relationships? How can you apply what you learned in this activity about comparing yourself to others to those situations or relationships?
17. How do you usually deal with frustration? How can you apply what you learned in this activity about handling frustration in those situations?
18. How can you improve the way you handle situations in which you are not in control and must depend on others for success? What did you learn in this activity you can apply to those situations?

Safety Concerns:

1. There are obvious concerns about tripping and falling with this quick-movement activity. These concerns are amplified if you try the variation that has the participants tie an ankle together.
2. Plastic lids can slip on some surfaces. Take care that the numbers participants are stepping on are stable and or fixed such that participants don't slip in their enthusiasm to quickly touch the numbers.

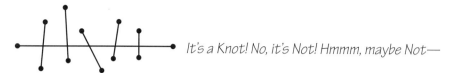

Name of Activity: Knot or Not

Type of Activity: *Deinhibitizer; Challenge/Initiative*

Grade Level: *First grade and up*

Size of Group: *1 to 20 or as many as can easily see the Knot— or not—*

Goal 1: Improve Communication and Relationship Skills

Objectives:

1A. Demonstrate understanding of and apply basic communication skills (e.g., recognizing nonverbal cues, delivering "I" messages)
1D. Express ideas clearly and constructively
1E. Listen actively to others
1F. Demonstrate willingness to trust others
1G. Develop skills for making and maintaining relationships
1H. Recognize and deal with peer pressure
1I. Use communication skills to resolve conflict
1J. Recognize the need for help and develop the ability to ask for it
1L. Develop skills for effectively participating in groups

Goal 3: Develop and Apply Problem-Solving and Decision-Making Skills

Objectives:

3B. Identify problems
3C. Demonstrate understanding of steps for solving problems and making decisions (gather information; explore alternatives and consequences; plan and take action)
3D. Evaluate decisions
3F. Apply decision-making skills to resolve conflicts
3G. Apply decision-making skills in life situations
3H. Demonstrate effective coping skills for dealing with problems
3I. Recognize when peer pressure is influencing decision making
3J. Develop ability to identify alternative methods for solving problems and achieving goals

Goal 6: Enhance Positive Attitudes and Skills Related to Learning

Objectives:

6C. Accept mistakes as part of the learning process
6G. Develop the ability to share knowledge
6H. Develop critical-thinking skills

Materials: Rope, string, webbing, yarn, or some other material that COULD be tied in a knot. We like to use rope or webbing and use 15 to 20 feet. However, you can also use string and have only 1 to 2 feet. If you use a smaller material, it may be harder (or more challenging depending upon how you think about it) for a larger group to see and judge whether there is a knot or not.

Preparation: Tie an overhand knot (the first part of tying your shoelaces), or don't, in the rope, string, or other material you are using. Arrange the rope or string in a pile (e.g., mess or tangle) on the floor with both ends of the rope extending out of the pile on opposite ends.

How to Play:

1. In this activity, the group has to decide whether, after fully extending the rope, there will be a knot in the rope or whether it will extend in a straight line without a knot. You obviously know because you either tied an overhand knot in the rope before arranging it in a pile, or you didn't.

2. Explain to the group that the task is for the group to decide whether there is a knot in the rope on the floor, or not.
3. Participants can inspect, but not touch, the rope.
4. After a set amount of time (you be the judge, based on your group, but shorter is almost always better) have the group vote on whether they think there is a knot in the rope, or not. We like to have them vote by moving to one side of the rope pile to indicate "knot" and the other side to indicate "not a knot."
5. After the vote, have two participants pull on the two extended ends of the rope until the rope is fully extended and the group can see whether in fact there was a knot, or not.

Variations:

1. One variation is to set a boundary around the rope pile. We often use 4 to 5 feet. The group must judge the rope pile and determine whether there is a knot or not from behind the boundary.
2. If a boundary is used, after the first vote you can let participants move inside the boundary to inspect the pile and then, with this new perspective, vote again.
3. Whether you use boundaries or not, after a first vote (or two), you can have two participants pull one of the ends of the rope just a bit. After the rope pile has been slightly diminished (because some of the rope is now extended away from the pile after being pulled by the two participants), have the participants drop the rope ends and have the group reinspect the new pile and vote again.
4. After the preceding step, or at any other time when participants might vote, instead of voting, ask them to see if they can come to consensus on whether there is a knot, or not.

Sample Personalization-Processing Questions:

1. How did you go about deciding whether there was a knot? How did the other members of the group decide? How important was generating ideas and brainstorming? What other problem-solving processes did the group members use? Which decision-making strategies appealed to you?
2. If you were pretty certain about whether there was a knot, did you try to influence the opinions of others in the group? If yes, what persuasive techniques did you use? Were there more effective ways for you to share your knowledge?
3. If other people expressed certainty about whether there was a knot, how did this affect your decision-making process? Did anyone try to persuade you to agree with their opinion?
4. Did these interactions feel like peer pressure? If yes, what part of the interactions felt like peer pressure? How did you cope with it?
5. How did you feel when you guessed correctly? How did you feel when you guessed incorrectly? How did you express those feelings? What did you tell yourself about yourself and/or your abilities when you guessed incorrectly?
6. Were you correct more often or incorrect more often? How did you define whether you were successful at this activity? If you were successful, how did you feel about that? If you were unsuccessful, how did you feel about that?
7. If the leader used the variations in which there was a boundary keeping you away from the rope, how did this affect your accuracy?
8. If the leader used the variation in which you got to move the rope a bit and vote again, how did this affect your accuracy?
9. How important was it for you to listen to the reasoning of other group members in the process of deciding whether there was a knot? Did their opinions affect your formation of your own opinion?
10. Did some of the interactions among group members feel like conflict to you? If yes, how did you handle the conflict? What were some ways you could have handled the conflict more effectively?
11. Did you communicate your ideas and feelings effectively? If so, how did you go about doing this? If not, what prevented you from doing this?
12. If you were feeling confused and couldn't decide how to vote, how comfortable were you asking for help from the other members of the group?

Sample Application-Processing Questions:

1. What are other situations or relationships in your life in which you need to make decisions about the accuracy of your perceptions? How can you apply what you learned in this activity in these situations?

2. What are other situations or relationships in your life in which others might try to influence your decisions? How can you apply what you learned in this activity in these situations?

3. What is your usual method of making decisions? How could you use what you learned in this activity to enhance your decision making?

4. Which of the methods for problem solving or decision making used by the members of this group would be useful in other situations in your life? How can you use them in these situations?

5. What are some other situations or relationships in which it might be useful for you to listen to others? How do you go about deciding whether to let yourself be influenced by listening to others?

6. How can you apply some of the methods of resolving conflicts that you learned/practiced in this activity in other situations?

7. How do you deal with situations in which you disagree with what the other members of a group decide? How can you apply what you learned in this activity to those situations?

8. What did you learn about your critical-thinking skills that you can apply to other situations in your life?

9. What are some situations in your life in which it is critical to share your knowledge with others? How do you feel when you get to share your knowledge with others?

10. How can you apply some of the methods that you learned/practiced in this activity for dealing with peer pressure or asking for help in other situations?

11. What are other situations or relationships in your life in which you need to make decisions about whether you are successful? How can you apply what you learned in this activity in these situations?

12. When you judge your performance as not being successful, how does this affect you? What do you tell yourself about yourself and/or your ability in those situations? What are some more positive ways for you to think about yourself and/or your abilities when you are not successful?

Safety Concerns: None—unless things get so heated in the discussion that someone tries to use the rope for something other than a knot. Never happened to us— but we're just saying—

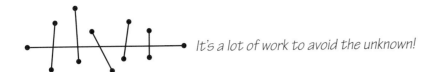

It's a lot of work to avoid the unknown!

Name of Activity: Known and Unknown

Type of Activity: *Icebreaker; Deinhibitizer*

Grade Level: *First grade and up*

Size of Group: *8 to 30, maybe more*

Goal 2: Increase Self-Awareness and Self-Acceptance

Objectives:

2A. Explore personal attitudes and values
2G. Recognize personal boundaries, rights, and privacy needs
2H. Identify personal and social roles

Goal 3: Develop and Apply Problem-Solving and Decision-Making Skills

Objectives:

3A. Set personal goals
3E. Manage change and transitions in everyday life
3H. Demonstrate effective coping skills for dealing with problems
3J. Develop ability to identify alternative methods for solving problems and achieving goals

Goal 5: Demonstrate Consistently Responsible Behavior

Objectives:

5D. Develop coping skills for dealing with stress
5E. Understand the need for self-discipline and self-control and how to exercise them

Materials: Open space

Preparation: None (isn't that a beautiful thing?)

How to Play:

1. This is a simple and quick game that involves some movement.
2. First, have each member of the group silently identify the person in the group he or she knows the very best (e.g., already friends with, seen around, chatted with before the group).
3. After each person can indicate that he or she has identified this person (to themselves and without disclosing who it is to you or the rest of the group), ask group members to think of that person as their Known (the person they know best in the group). We often ask participants to raise their hands if they "have their Known."
4. Next ask each member of the group to silently identify the person he or she knows the least well in the group.
5. Again, after each person can indicate that he or she has identified this person (only to themselves and not disclosing the identity to the group), ask group members to think of that person as their Unknown. Again, we often ask participants to raise their hands if they "have their Unknown."
6. Once each participant has identified his or her Known and Unknown, explain that the object of the activity for all participants is to, without disclosing who their Known and Unknown are, move around the space attempting to keep their Known between themselves and their Unknown.
7. This is a walking activity, and participants try to move such that their Known is always in the line between themselves and their Unknown. Of course, one of the challenges is that each person's Known and Unknown have Knowns and Unknowns of their own who are all moving

to try to accomplish the same task. As a result, it as an ongoing challenge to keep your Known between you and your Unknown.

Sample Personalization-Processing Questions:

1. How did you decide who was your Known and who was your Unknown?
2. How did your choices reflect your ideas about friendship? How did your choices reflect your values?
3. Did you wonder whose Known you were? Whose Unknown you were? If you found out, how did you feel about it?
4. How did you feel when either your Known or your Unknown moved?
5. How did you deal with the transitions involved in the constant movement of this game?
6. What strategies did you use to keep your Known between you and your Unknown?
7. How did you judge whether your strategy was working? If it wasn't working, how did you generate a new strategy that would be more effective?
8. On a 1 to 10 scale, how stressful was this activity for you? What made it stressful? Where did you feel the stress in your body? What could you have done to make the activity less stressful for you?
9. Why did you need to exercise self-control and self-discipline in this activity? How did that go for you? What were some ways you could have increased your application of self-control and self-discipline during this activity?
10. What did you learn about yourself during this activity?

Sample Application-Processing Questions:

1. How do you usually decide whether someone is known (whether you feel close to that person)? How do you usually decide whether someone is unknown (whether you feel distant from that person)?
2. How do you go about deciding whether a person is someone with whom you would like to make friends? How does this process reflect your attitudes and values?
3. When you have decided you would like to be friends with someone, how do you go about making friends with that person?
4. What is your attitude toward transitions?
5. What kinds of transitions do you usually have to make in your life? How do you usually go about making transitions? How can you apply what you learned in this activity about you and transitions to these other situations?
6. What are some other situations in which you feel as though you are constantly moving (or the situation in constantly in flux)? How can you apply what you learned in this activity about yourself to these other situations?
7. What are some other situations or relationships that you find stressful? How can you apply what you learned in this activity about dealing with stress in these other situations?
8. What are some other situations or relationships in which you must exercise self-control and self-discipline? How can you apply what you learned in this activity about dealing with stress in these other situations?

Safety Concerns: None, as long as folks are WALKING.

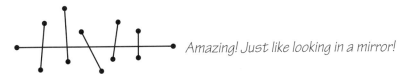

Amazing! Just like looking in a mirror!

Name of Activity: Mirror Mirror

Type of Activity: Icebreaker

Grade Level: First grade and up

Size of Group: 8 to 100, maybe more—need an even number for partners—or YOU can play! We do!

Goal 1: Improve Communication and Relationship Skills

Objectives:

1A.   Demonstrate understanding of and apply basic communication skills (e.g., recognizing nonverbal cues, delivering "I" messages)

1G.   Develop skills for making and maintaining relationships

Goal 2: Increase Self-Awareness and Self-Acceptance

Objective:

2H.   Identify personal and social roles

Goal 4: Increase Understanding and Valuing of Diversity

Objectives:

4A.   Recognize and appreciate individual differences

4B.   Develop an understanding and appreciation of own culture

4C.   Demonstrate respect for others as both individuals and members of different cultural groups

4D.   Acknowledge and appreciate similarities and differences across cultures and/or groups of people who have physical or learning differences

Goal 5: Demonstrate Consistently Responsible Behavior

Objectives:

5B.   Recognize whether behavior is appropriate and responsible

5C.   Act in an appropriate and responsible manner

5D.   Develop coping skills for dealing with stress

5E.   Understand the need for self-discipline and self-control and how to exercise them

5G.   Demonstrate respect for alternate perspectives

Goal 6: Enhance Positive Attitudes and Skills Related to Learning

Objectives:

6A.   Develop feeling of competence and confidence as a learner

6B.   Take pride in accomplishments

6C.   Accept mistakes as part of the learning process

6E.   Recognize that effort and persistence enhance learning

Materials: None

Preparation: None

How to Play:

1.   Have participants find a partner. It is often fun if it is someone they don't know terribly well.

2. Ask participants to stand facing their partners.
3. Each pair must determine who will go first.
4. This person is the initial Leader in the activity.
5. Explain that the Leader in each pair will engage in some physical movement (you might want to model something fun like waving one hand or turning to the side), and the other participant in the pair is to mimic that movement so that it looks like the mirror image of the Leader's actions.
6. Interestingly, you are asking the Follower in each pair to actually do the exact opposite of the Leader. For instance, if the Leader raises his or her right arm, the Follower—in order to mirror the Leader—actually raises his or her left arm (because they are facing each other). (This is likely overexplaining—but hey, we're PhDs.)
7. Ask the participants to complete the activity in silence.
8. Yell "Go!" and watch the fun.
9. After a brief time (judged by your assessment of how much fun the participants are having—and how much energy they have for the activity), have the participants stop and switch roles.
10. After both partners have acted as a Mirror to their respective partners, ask them to engage in the same activity EXCEPT that followers should do the opposite of their partners.
11. Literally you're asking followers to do exactly the same thing as the leaders (when the leader raises his or her right hand, the follower raises his or her right hand—doing the exact same thing—but because they are standing facing each other, it looks like the opposite). (Sorry, that pesky PhD thing again.)

Sample Personalization-Processing Questions:

1. How did it feel to be the Leader? What did you like about it? What didn't you like about it? How could you get more comfortable with leading others?
2. How did it feel to be the Follower? What did you like about it? What didn't you like about it? How could you get more comfortable with following the lead of others?
3. How was it for you when you transitioned from being the leader to being the follower (or vice versa)? How did you handle these transitions? Were there some things you could have done to make the transitions smoother?
4. How was it for you when you transitioned from mirroring your partner into doing the opposite of what your partner did? How did you handle these transitions? Were there some things you could have done to make the transitions smoother?
5. As time passed, did you feel more competent as a leader? As a follower?
6. How did you feel as you got the following right? How did you silently communicate those feelings to your partner?
7. On a 1 to 10 scale, how stressful was leading for you? What made it stressful? Where did you feel the stress in your body? What could you have done to make the activity less stressful for you?
8. On a 1 to 10 scale, how stressful was following for you? What made it stressful? Where did you feel the stress in your body? What could you have done to make the activity less stressful for you?
9. Why did you need to exercise self-control and self-discipline in this activity? How did that go for you? What were some ways you could have increased your self-control and self-discipline during this activity?
10. How were the movements you did when you were the leader different from the movements that your partner did when he or she was the leader? How were the movements you and your partner chose different from the movements that others in the group chose?
11. Did you notice any patterns across the members in the group related to the kinds of movement that people chose? What were those patterns? Were those patterns related in any way to the culture of those leading at the time?
12. Did you notice any stereotypes you were holding about certain people in this process? How did your holding those stereotypes affect how you interpreted the way they moved?
13. What were your responsibilities to your partner in this activity? How did you decide what your responsibilities were?
14. Did you honor those responsibilities to your partner? If yes, what kinds of things did you do that you felt were responsible? How did you make sure your behavior was responsible? If no,

what kinds of things did you do that you felt were not responsible? What kept you from being more responsible during this activity?

15. How could you tell whether your partner perceived your behaviors as responsible? What kinds of feedback did you get from your partner about whether you were being responsible during this activity? How did you react when you got this kind of feedback?

16. If your partner was being irresponsible in his or her leading, how did you go about choosing whether to follow his or her movements?

17. If you had trouble duplicating your partner's movements, what did you tell yourself about yourself and your ability to move? If it was easy to duplicate your partner's movements, what did you tell yourself?

18. What did you learn about yourself during this activity?

Sample Application-Processing Questions:

1. What are some situations or relationships in your life in which you are the leader? How do you feel about being the leader? What did you learn in this activity that could help you be more comfortable with being a leader?

2. What are some situations or relationships in your life in which you are the follower? How do you feel about being the follower? What did you learn in this activity that could help you be more comfortable with being a follower?

3. What are some situations in your life in which you must handle transitions (in roles, in behaviors, in priorities, in responsibilities, etc.)? What did you learn in this activity that could help you be more comfortable with making transitions?

4. What are the rules (spoken or unspoken) about being a leader or a follower in your family? In your culture?

5. What are some other situations in which you have noticed differences in people's comfort levels with being a leader? Being a follower? What were the differences that you noticed? If someone else has different rules than you do about being a leader or a follower, how can you handle these differences in an appropriate, respectful way?

6. What are the rules (spoken or unspoken) about being fully expressive with your body in your family? In your culture?

7. What are some other situations in which you have noticed differences in people's comfort levels about being fully expressive with their bodies? What were the differences that you noticed? If someone else has different rules than you do about being fully expressive with their bodies, how can you handle this in an appropriate, respectful way?

8. What are some situations or relationships in which you feel that it is really important to act in a responsible manner? How do you handle these situations or relationships?

9. What are some times when you do not act as responsibly as you think you should? What do you think keeps you from being more responsible in those situations? How could you handle those situations differently in the future?

10. How do you feel when you get feedback that you are not acting in a responsible manner? How do you react to this feedback? How is your reaction affected by who it is that is giving the feedback? By the way the feedback is delivered?

11. What are some other situations in your life in which it is important to exercise self-control and self-discipline? How can you apply what you learned during this activity about your ability to exercise self-control and self-discipline to these situations?

12. What are some other situations in your life in which a person's willingness to act in a responsible manner can affect your ability to trust him or her?

13. What are some other situations in your life in which you could notice and celebrate your own uniqueness? Your successes?

14. What are some situations in which you would choose not to follow a leader who was acting in an irresponsible manner? How would you handle those situations? How can you apply what you learned in this activity to those situations?

Safety Concerns: None, as long as leaders don't get too carried away in their physical actions—

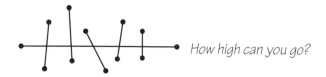 *How high can you go?*

Name of Activity: Moon Ball

Type of Activity: *Deinhibitizer; Challenge/Initiative*

Grade Level: *First grade and up (surprisingly effective with adult groups)*

Size of Group: *5 to 30, maybe more*

Goal 1: Improve Communication and Relationship Skills

Objectives:

1A. Demonstrate understanding of and apply basic communication skills (e.g., recognizing nonverbal cues, delivering "I" messages)
1B. Express feelings clearly and constructively
1C. Recognize and accept the feelings of others
1D. Express ideas clearly and constructively
1E. Listen actively to others
1G. Develop skills for making and maintaining relationships
1H. Recognize and deal with peer pressure
1I. Use communication skills to resolve conflict
1J. Recognize the need for help and develop the ability to ask for it
1K. Recognize and verbalize needs and wishes
1L. Develop skills for effectively participating in groups

Goal 3: Develop and Apply Problem-Solving and Decision-Making Skills

Objectives:

3A. Set personal goals
3B. Identify problems
3C. Demonstrate understanding of steps for solving problems and making decisions (gather information; explore alternatives and consequences; plan and take action)
3D. Evaluate decisions
3E. Manage change and transitions in everyday life
3F. Apply decision-making skills to resolve conflicts
3G. Apply decision-making skills in life situations
3H. Demonstrate effective coping skills for dealing with problems
3I. Recognize when peer pressure is influencing decision making
3J. Develop ability to identify alternative methods for solving problems and achieving goals

Goal 6: Enhance Positive Attitudes and Skills Related to Learning

Objectives:

6B. Take pride in accomplishments
6C. Accept mistakes as part of the learning process
6E. Recognize that effort and persistence enhance learning
6F. Demonstrate dependability and initiative
6G. Develop the ability to share knowledge
6H. Develop critical-thinking skills

Materials: Open space and an inflated beach ball

Preparation: Inflate the beach ball.

How to Play:

1. This is a simple game of keeping the beach ball in the air.
2. Using volleyball-like techniques, the participants work together to keep the ball in the air.
3. Like volleyball, no participant can hit the ball two consecutive times.
4. Unlike volleyball, each time a participant hits the ball in the air, the group can add to their count of hits.
5. When/if the beach ball hits the ground, the count begins at 1 again.

Variations:

1. Have the group pick a goal for how many hits they can complete without letting the ball hit the ground.
2. Have the group complete the task in silence (perhaps with you doing the counting).

Sample Personalization-Processing Questions:

1. How did the members of the group work together as a team? Why was it important to work as a team?
2. How did you feel when the group worked together as a team? How did you feel when the group was not working together well? How did you express your feelings to the rest of the group?
3. How did you feel when someone dropped the ball and the group had to start over? How did you feel when someone hit the ball twice and the group had to start over? How did you express those feelings to the group? What were some ways you could have expressed your feelings to the group more clearly and constructively?
4. Did you have some ideas about how the members of the group could improve their ability to work together as a team? How did you express your ideas to the group? What were some ways you could have expressed your ideas to the group more clearly and constructively?
5. How did the group members decide how many hits were enough? (How did the group define *success*?) Were you in agreement with the other members of the group about this? If not, how did you handle that?
6. What did you do to contribute to the success of the group? How did you feel about your contribution?
7. Did the members of the group generate ideas on how to be more effective in keeping the ball up? If yes, how did the members of the group go about this process? If no, how did you feel about it when the group was not very effective at keeping the ball up?
8. If the group talked strategy, did everyone feel heard as the group was coming up with a more effective technique of keeping the ball up? How did it feel when you were heard by other members of the group? If you didn't feel heard, what was that like for you? If you had wanted to be heard by the other members of the group, what could you have done differently to make sure that you were heard?
9. Did you communicate your ideas and feelings effectively? If so, how did you go about doing this? If not, what prevented you from doing this?
10. What process did the members of the group use to determine the best way to keep the ball up? How did the group members decide whether a strategy was working? If a strategy wasn't working, how did the group members deal with that? How did you go about developing an alternative strategy when something wasn't working?
11. How did you decide whether to cooperate or not? How did your attitudes about cooperation influence what happened in the group? What about the attitudes of other group members?
12. How could you tell whether you needed help from other group members? What did you do when you needed help? How did you ask for help when you recognized you needed it?
13. If you were one of the people who dropped the ball and caused the group to have to start over, how did you feel about this? What did you tell yourself about your competence when this happened? What did you tell yourself about other group members when this happened? What did you communicate to the rest of the group when mistakes happened?
14. If you never dropped the ball how did you feel about those who did? How did you express your feelings to the group?
15. How did you treat the person who dropped the ball? Were there better, more appropriate ways to communicate about your thoughts and feelings when this happened?

16. What was your level of stress during this activity? How did your stress level change as the number of hits grew? How did your stress level change if your group could not seem to get very many hits in a row? What strategies did you use to cope with the stress involved in this activity?

17. When members of the group disagreed on strategies for keeping the ball up, did you interpret the interactions as conflict? If you did, how did you feel about the conflict? What did you do about your feelings? How did the group members resolve the conflict? What would have been some other ways to do this?

18. In what ways did peer pressure affect the process of keeping the ball up? How did the members of your group handle the peer pressure?

19. What personal positive traits and talents did you bring to this process, and how did you use them to help in keeping the ball up?

20. If you were feeling discouraged in this process, how did you deal with that? What did you tell yourself to motivate yourself to continue? If other group members were feeling discouraged, how did you interact with them about their discouragement?

21. How did you feel about it when the group kept the ball up for a long time? How did you communicate those feelings to the rest of the group?

22. What impact did persistence and effort have on the group's ability to keep the ball up?

23. If you did the activity in silence, how was that different than being able to talk?

24. If there were participants with physical challenges, how did the group deal with those?

Sample Application-Processing Questions:

1. How do you define success in other situations in your life? How can you apply what you learned in this activity about yourself and the way you think and feel about success to other situations in your life?

2. What are other situations or relationships in your life in which it feels as though you must keep a ball in the air? What resources do you have to help you deal with these situations?

3. What are some other situations in your life in which you must have cooperation and help (work as a team) to be successful? How do you deal with these situations? How do you elicit cooperation and help? What did you learn in this activity about working as a team that you can apply to those situations?

4. Which of the methods for managing stress that you or the members of your group used can be helpful in other situations in your life? How can you use them?

5. What are some other situations in which you might need to ask for help? How can you go about recognizing that you need help and asking for it?

6. What are some other situations or relationships in which it might be important for you to be heard? How can you go about making sure that you are heard in those situations?

7. How can you apply some of the methods for communicating about feelings and ideas, encouraging cooperation, solving problems, and/or appropriately resolving conflicts that you learned/practiced in this activity in other situations?

8. How can you apply what you learned about dealing with mistakes in other situations? Dealing with negative self-talk? Encouraging persistence and flexibility? Dealing with peer pressure? Dealing with stress?

9. What did you learn about your critical-thinking skills that you can apply to other situations in your life?

10. What are some situations in your life in which sharing information with others is important? How can you get better at presenting information in a way that encourages others to listen and use the information?

Safety Concerns: None, as long as folks are WALKING. Enthusiastic running after the ball can lead to inadvertent participant collisions.

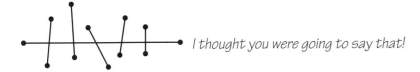
I thought you were going to say that!

Name of Activity: Negotiation Square

Type of Activity: *Deinhibitizer, Challenge/Initiative*

Grade Level: *Fourth grade and up*

Size of Group: *8 to 100*

Goal 1: Improve Communication and Relationship Skills

Objectives:

1A.   Demonstrate understanding of and apply basic communication skills (e.g., recognizing nonverbal cues, delivering "I" messages)
1B.   Express feelings clearly and constructively
1C.   Recognize and accept the feelings of others
1D.   Express ideas clearly and constructively
1E.   Listen actively to others
1H.   Recognize and deal with peer pressure
1I.   Use communication skills to resolve conflict
1J.   Recognize the need for help and develop the ability to ask for it
1K.   Recognize and verbalize needs and wishes
1L.   Develop skills for effectively participating in groups

Goal 3: Develop and Apply Problem-Solving and Decision-Making Skills

Objectives:

3A.   Set personal goals
3B.   Identify problems
3C.   Demonstrate understanding of steps for solving problems and making decisions (gather information; explore alternatives and consequences; plan and take action)
3D.   Evaluate decisions
3F.   Apply decision-making skills to resolve conflicts
3G.   Apply decision-making skills in life situations
3H.   Demonstrate effective coping skills for dealing with problems
3I.   Recognize when peer pressure is influencing decision making
3J.   Develop ability to identify alternative methods for solving problems and achieving goals

Goal 6: Enhance Positive Attitudes and Skills Related to Learning

Objectives:

6A.   Develop feeling of competence and confidence as a learner
6B.   Take pride in accomplishments
6C.   Accept mistakes as part of the learning process
6D.   Apply time management and task management strategies
6E.   Recognize that effort and persistence enhance learning
6G.   Develop the ability to share knowledge
6H.   Develop critical-thinking skills

Materials: None

Preparation: None

How to Play:

1. Have the group split up into four roughly equal subgroups.
2. Explain that each group should arrange themselves in a line so that the four groups make up the sides of a square (or the rough equivalent if the groups are not equal).
3. After the square has been formed (and the groups have a sense of what the square will be like, where they should stand, etc.), have the groups take a step or two back and huddle up so that the members of each subgroup can see and hear one another. At this point the large group should be in four smaller subgroup huddles, each representing a side of the square.
4. The task for each of the subgroups (now huddled up) is to decide on a sound, word, or phrase they would like to say together and an accompanying gesture. You may need to prompt the group to get the brainstorming started. You can also explain that this can be a cheer, an expression of the group, or a hope for the day.
5. After each group has separately decided on their own cheer/sound and gesture, have the four groups re-form the square.
6. Explain to the group that each subgroup (side of the square) will now have a chance to show their sound/gesture to the other three groups.
7. In whatever order you'd like (after all, you're the leader so it's your world) have each group show off its sound/gesture by having all of the members of the subgroup (side of the square) make the sound (or say the word[s]) and make the gesture all at the same time.
8. After each group shows off their sound/gesture, we like to have the other three groups applaud. Then, we like to have all of the groups do the sound/gesture at the same time. In this way the one subgroup is teaching the other three groups their sound/gesture.
9. Continue in whatever order you'd like (it is, after all, your world) so that all four groups have shown off their sound/gesture, and the entire group has practiced all of the sounds/gestures of all the groups.
10. After all the sounds/gestures have been shown off and practiced, have the subgroups (sides of the square) huddle up again.
11. Explain to the subgroups that the object of the activity at this point is, without talking or communicating with the other subgroups, to simultaneously decide to all do the same sound/gesture at the same time. That is, each subgroup can choose to repeat their own sound/gesture or adopt the sound/gesture of another group. Note that all members of each subgroup need to do the same sound/gesture. It is a subgroup decision that may need to be negotiated.
12. After each subgroup has decided which sound/gesture they are going to do (their own or that of another subgroup) they should re-form their side of the square.
13. When the square is complete, indicating that each subgroup (or side of the square) has decided which sound/gesture to do, explain that you will count to three and on the four beat (e.g., 1, 2, 3, X) each subgroup should make the sound/gesture they decided on.
14. With much fanfare, count one, two, three, and on the four beat all the groups should make their sound/gesture with the goal of, without having communicated across groups, all making the same sound and gesture.
15. If the groups in fact do make the same sound/gesture, you are obviously an amazingly gifted counselor/therapist/facilitator, and we bow to your superior skill and ability. We suggest you declare victory and have a celebration. We, however, have never had this happen.
16. If all four groups do not make the same sound/gesture, ask the subgroups (sides of the square) to rehuddle and decide what sound/gesture to do in another round. Groups can stick to their guns and do the same sound/gesture or can switch to any of the others.
17. After each subgroup has decided which sound/gesture they will make this time, have them re-form the square and try again.
18. Count one, two, three, have the subgroups make their sound/gesture on the four beat, and see where you are—
19. Continue with these rounds until you get consensus on the sound/gesture (exemplified by the simultaneous sound/gesture—typically followed by much rejoicing) or until you think the activity has run its course (e.g., three groups doing the same sound/gesture and the one other repeatedly doing a different sound/gesture, indicating that consensus is unlikely without some higher order diplomacy, which is likely to be beyond the time frame you have allowed).

Variations:

Sometimes for fun, after each group has shown off their sound/gesture for the first time, we conduct a sound/gesture symphony. We stand in the middle of the square and explain that when we point at a group they should make their own sound/gesture. We typically start by simply going around the square in one direction, pointing at each group so they get the feel of it. Then we feel free to run wild (which is not out of character for us) and point at various groups at various times (sometimes having a group repeat their sound/gesture two or three times in a row), all in the service of creating a sound/gesture symphony. We usually end with a quick flourish and encourage applause. Groups often find this fun, and we always do.

Sample Personalization-Processing Questions:

1. What was fun for you about this activity? What was frustrating about it?
2. How did your subgroup make up your sound? Did everyone have input into the process of choosing the sound? As all of the groups demonstrated their sounds, did you compare your subgroup's sound to the others? What impact did that comparison have on you? (Did you still like your sound or did you want a new one?)
3. How did the members of your subgroup decide which sound to make when all the subgroups joined the square? How did your subgroup come to a consensus about what sound to make? How did you decide whether a strategy for picking the sound to make was working? What did the members of your subgroup do if they decided a strategy wasn't working?
4. How did you feel when your subgroup made a mistake and got a guess wrong? How did you express those feelings? What did you tell yourself about yourself and/or the other members of your subgroup when you guessed incorrectly?
5. How did you feel when your subgroup made a sound that matched one or more of the other subgroups? How did you express those feelings to the group? What did you tell yourself about yourself and/or the other members of your subgroup when you guessed correctly?
6. If you were pretty certain about what sound to make, did you try to influence the opinions of others in the group? If yes, what persuasive techniques did you use? What were some more effective or respectful ways for you to share your knowledge?
7. If other people in your subgroup expressed certainty about what sound to make, how did this effect your decision-making process? Did anyone try to persuade you to agree with their opinion? How did it feel?
8. Did these interactions feel like peer pressure? If yes, what part of the interactions felt like peer pressure? How did you cope with it?
9. Was your subgroup correct more often or incorrect more often? How did you define whether you were successful at this activity? If you were successful, how did you feel about that? If you were unsuccessful, how did you feel about that?
10. How did the members of your subgroup apply the learning from earlier turns as the game progressed?
11. When did you recognize that part of the process of successfully predicting what the other subgroups would do was to think like them? What were some methods your subgroup used to take the perspective of other subgroups? Why was this important?
12. Did some of the interactions between group members feel like conflict to you? If yes, how did you handle the conflict? What were some ways you could have handled the conflict more effectively?
13. How did you apply your critical-thinking skills in this activity? What were some ways you could have used your critical-thinking skills more effectively?
14. What did you do to contribute to the success of your subgroup? The entire group?
15. Did everyone feel heard as the various subgroups tried to develop strategies for predicting the sound that other subgroups would make? How did it feel when you were heard by other members of the group? What did you do to try to make sure that you were heard by the other members of the group?
16. If you didn't feel heard, what was that like for you? If you had wanted to be heard by the other members of the group, what could you have done differently to make sure that you were heard?
17. Did you communicate your ideas and feelings effectively? If so, how did you go about doing this? If not, what prevented you from doing this?

1. As you were playing the game, did it feel really important that your subgroup predict the sound that the other subgroups would make? Was it really important that you did this? What do you think about the fact that it seemed important at the time, but might not have really been important?

2. What are some times in school when you get worried about something that might not really be important but you think it is at the time? At home? In other situations?

3. What strategies can you use to determine whether something is really important? What are some ways you can get better at deciding whether something is really important?

4. What are other situations or relationships in your life in which others might try to influence your decisions? How can you apply what you learned in this activity in these situations?

5. What is your usual method of making decisions? How could you use what you learned in this activity to enhance your decision making?

6. Which of the methods for problem solving or decision making used by the members of this group would be useful in other situations in your life? How can you use them in these situations?

7. What are some other situations or relationships in which it might be useful for you to listen to others? How do you go about deciding whether to let yourself be influenced by listening to others?

8. How can you apply some of the methods of resolving conflicts that you learned/practiced in this activity in other situations?

9. How do you deal with situations in which you are in a group that must come to some kind of consensus? How can you apply what you learned in this activity to those situations?

10. What did you learn about your critical-thinking skills that you can apply to other situations in your life?

11. What are some situations in your life in which it is important to share your knowledge with others? How do you feel when you get to share your knowledge with others?

12. How can you apply some of the methods that you learned/practiced in this activity for dealing with peer pressure in other situations? Dealing with stress? Learning from mistakes? Recognizing that effort and persistence enhance learning?

13. What are other situations or relationships in your life in which you need to make decisions about whether you are successful? How can you apply what you learned in this activity in these situations?

14. When you judge your performance as not being successful, how does this affect you? What do you tell yourself about yourself and/or your ability in those situations? What are some more positive ways for you to think about yourself and/or your abilities when you are not successful?

15. What are some other situations or relationships in which you compare yourself to others? What has the impact of those comparisons been on you and/or your relationships? How can you apply what you learned in this activity about comparing yourself to others to those situations or relationships?

16. How do you usually deal with frustration? How can you apply what you learned in this activity about handling frustration in those situations?

Safety Concerns: None

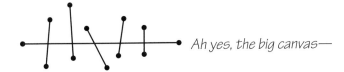

Ah yes, the big canvas—

Name of Activity: Paint Your Name

Type of Activity: *Icebreaker; Deinhibitizer*

Grade Level: *Second grade and up—particularly funny with adults*

Size of Group: *8 to 30, maybe more—most fun in a circle*

Goal 1: Improve Communication and Relationship Skills

Objectives:

    1H.   Recognize and deal with peer pressure
    1K.   Recognize and verbalize needs and wishes

Goal 2: Increase Self-Awareness and Self-Acceptance

Objectives:

    2B.   Identify and acknowledge personal positive traits, talents, and accomplishments
    2E.   Appreciate own uniqueness
    2G.   Recognize personal boundaries, rights, and privacy needs

Goal 4: Increase Understanding and Valuing of Diversity

Objectives:

    4A.   Recognize and appreciate individual differences
    4B.   Develop an understanding and appreciation of own culture

Goal 6: Enhance Positive Attitudes and Skills Related to Learning

Objective:

    6B.   Take pride in accomplishments

Materials: Open space for participants to move

Preparation: None

How to Play:

1. This is a simple and quick activity that involves some stretching and movement. Participants should be able to spell their names. If they are old enough to be able to write in cursive, that is a plus, but it isn't necessary.
2. Have the participants form a circle.
3. Explain to participants that the task is to, using their right hand (even if they are left-handed), write their name in the air as largely as they can. We always model reaching high into the air (up on tiptoes) and down to our knees to form an example letter or two. This lets participants know what we mean by *largely*.
4. Also explain that participants should move around in the circle (to the right—assuming your writing in a Latin-based language) so that the letters in the air are next to each other rather than on top of each other (which would be the case if you just stood in one place—very hard to read that way).
5. We often ask participants to imagine signing the world's largest painting or an amazingly big check.
6. On the word *go,* have everyone (we generally participate) write his or her name at the same time, pretending to write each letter as they move to their right around the circle.

7. After each person is done (note that the circle may have to keep moving even after some participants are done writing because others have longer names and/or have chosen to include their full middle or maiden names also), invite the group to write their names again, this time using their left hands.

8. Finally, after writing with both hands, ask participants to imagine placing the pen or paint brush in their navels and use their belly-button writing instrument to write their name one final time. Frankly, almost too funny—but not quite.

Sample Personalization-Processing Questions:

1. How did you feel about being so fully expressive with your body? How did you feel about doing something this silly? How did your feelings change with the different placements of the pen or paint brush? How did the fact that everybody was looking silly together affect your feelings?

2. Was the pace the group moved in the circle comfortable for you? What did you do if it wasn't? How did you let others know what you wanted or needed in terms of the pace of movement of the circle?

3. Did you notice any kind of peer pressure in doing this activity (for instance, moving faster because others in the circle wanted you to speed up, fear that others would tease you if you were fully expressive with your body, etc.)? If you felt any peer pressure, how did you deal with it?

4. Did you ever feel uncomfortable because someone was too close to you or invading your personal space? How did you deal with this?

5. Did you ever get feedback that you might be invading someone else's personal space? How did you deal with this?

6. How did the way you signed your name express who you are? How was the way you signed your name unique?

7. What did you notice about differences among the group members in the way they approached this activity?

8. What are the rules (spoken or unspoken) in your family about being silly in public? In your culture? Which of these rules are rules that do not fit for you? How do you handle this?

9. What are some accomplishments of which you are proud? How do you express this pride?

10. What are the rules (spoken or unspoken) about taking pride in your accomplishments in your family? In your culture? Which of these rules are rules that do not fit for you? How do you handle this?

11. What are the rules (spoken or unspoken) about being fully expressive with your body in your family? In your culture? Which of these rules are rules that do not fit for you? How do you handle this?

Sample Application-Processing Questions:

1. What are some things you might do in your life that would warrant having a flamboyant signing ceremony?

2. What are some situations and/or relationships in your life in which you get a chance to express your uniqueness? How do you express this uniqueness?

3. Are you satisfied with the number of opportunities to express your uniqueness? If not, how could you increase these opportunities?

4. What are some other situations in your life in which you might experience peer pressure to be silly or not be silly? What are some other situations in which you might experience peer pressure to hide your uniqueness or accomplishments? How do you/will you deal with these situations? How could you apply what you learned during this game to these situations?

5. What are some other situations in your life in which it would be important to ask for what you need and want? What did you learn from this game that you could apply in situations in which it would be important to ask for what you need and want?

6. What are some other situations in your life in which it would be important to recognize and maintain your personal boundaries, rights, and privacy needs? What did you learn from this game that you could apply in these situations?

7. What are some other situations in your life in which you do not necessarily follow the rules of your family or culture? How do you handle those situations? How can you apply what you learned in this activity to these situations?

Safety Concerns: None, as long as their imaginary writing utensil isn't too sharp.

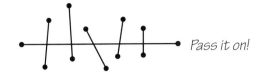
Pass it on!

Name of Activity: Pass the Tire

Type of Activity: Icebreaker; Deinhibitizer

Grade Level: Kindergarten and up

Size of Group: 6 to 20

Goal 1: Improve Communication and Relationship Skills

Objectives:

1D.   Express ideas clearly and constructively
1E.   Listen actively to others
1F.   Demonstrate willingness to trust others
1H.   Recognize and deal with peer pressure
1J.   Recognize the need for help and develop the ability to ask for it
1L.   Develop skills for effectively participating in groups

Goal 2: Increase Self-Awareness and Self-Acceptance

Objectives:

2C.   Develop ability to recognize negative self-talk
2D.   Develop skills in replacing negative self-talk with positive self-talk
2F.   Develop positive attitudes toward self
2G.   Recognize personal boundaries, rights, and privacy needs

Goal 3: Develop and Apply Problem-Solving and Decision-Making Skills

Objectives:

3H.   Demonstrate effective coping skills for dealing with problems
3I.   Recognize when peer pressure is influencing decision making
3J.   Develop ability to identify alternative methods for solving problems and achieving goals

Goal 4: Increase Understanding and Valuing of Diversity

Objectives:

4A.   Recognize and appreciate individual differences
4E.   Recognize how stereotypes can affect interpersonal relationships and attitudes toward others

Goal 5: Demonstrate Consistently Responsible Behavior

Objectives:

5D.   Develop coping skills for dealing with stress
5E.   Understand the need for self-discipline and self-control and how to exercise them

Goal 6: Enhance Positive Attitudes and Skills Related to Learning

Objective:

6B.   Take pride in accomplishments

Materials: Old bicycle tire inner tube

Preparation: None

How to Play:

1. Have everyone form a circle facing inward and holding hands.
2. At one point in the circle, break the circle and have one person put his or her arm through the inside of the tire inner tube. Have that person rejoin hands with the person next to him or her.
3. Explain to the members of the group that the object of this activity is to pass the tire inner tube around the entire circle without letting go of hands.
4. To accomplish the task, each participant will have to pass his or her body through the inner tube so that the tube gets to his or her opposite hand.
5. We like to require that whoever is passing the tire inner tube over themselves talk about themselves during the transition!
6. Note that even though participants can't let go of each others' hands, they can help the participant who is trying to pass through the tire inner tube.

Variations:

1. Make the tube smaller by tying a knot in the tube. Note that the smaller the tube the more challenging the activity.
2. To make it easier, you can use a hula hoop instead of a tire inner tube. However, a tube gives you much more flexibility in that you can adjust the size of the tube (by tying or adjusting a knot in the tube), and it stretches (the size might seem small to participants, but it will stretch around any size person—we have seen a group get a person in a wheelchair through a stretched tire inner tube). In addition, old tubes can often be obtained free from local bike shops.
3. Have each individual answer a question as he or she works his or her way through the tube.
4. Use two tire inner tubes and start one going in each direction and see where the tubes meet.
5. Instead of using a tire inner tube, use a long piece of 1–inch tubular webbing (10 to 20 feet long). Tie the webbing into a large loop, and then place another knot in the middle of the large loop, creating two smaller loops of equal size. Place the two loops over one person's arm. Instruct the group that one of the loops is to be passed around in a clockwise fashion and the other loop is to be passed around counterclockwise. At some point, the loops will cross over one another and then move around the circle.[1]
6. If you have more than one circle of participants, you can bring the circles together in a concentric way by taking a large loop (using 8 to 10 feet of 1–inch tubular webbing) and making a loop and then placing the loop over two different people's arms in two different groups. The task now becomes for two people (one from each circle) to go through the loop together. In this scenario, if you have more than two groups you could link all groups together in this manner. (Every group would be connected to two other groups.)
7. Have one person sit in a chair and have the group help this person through the tire inner tube without standing up. Players may lend assistance to others in the group.

Sample Personalization-Processing Questions:

1. What was your initial reaction when the leader described the activity?
2. What did you think about your ability to get your whole body through the tire inner tube? If you were pessimistic about your chances of getting through the tube, how did that affect your chances of getting through it? If you were optimistic about your chances of getting through the tube, how did that affect your chances of getting through it?
3. How might people's images of their bodies affect their reaction to this activity? How did your body image affect your reaction to this activity?
4. How did you feel about holding hands with the other people in the group? If you didn't want to hold hands, how did you handle it?
5. What about this activity required you to trust others? How was that experience for you?
6. How did you decide if you needed help getting through the tire inner tube? If you had to ask for help from others to get through the tube, how did you feel about that? How did you go about asking for help? How could you have gotten more comfortable with asking for help?

[1]*Note.* Adapted from Cain, J., & Smith, T. (2002). *The book of raccoon circles.* Dubuque, IA: Kendall Hunt.

7. How did it feel to be the center of attention, going through the tire inner tube and talking about yourself? What was hardest for you—having everybody in the group listen to you or having everybody in the group watching you go through the tube? What was hard about it? Why was that harder for you?

8. How did being the center of attention affect your stress level? How did you deal with it if you felt stressed out?

9. How did you decide what to tell the group about yourself? What kinds of things did you say (positive things, negative things, accomplishments, mistakes, funny things, etc.)?

10. How were the things you talked about different from the things that others told about themselves? What did you notice about your uniqueness?

11. How were the things you told about yourself similar to the things that other people told about themselves? What did you notice about what you had in common with others in the group?

12. Did you have any stereotypes that affected your perspective on certain people going through the inner tube? What was the impact of you holding those stereotypes?

13. How did standing so close to others and holding their hands affect how you felt about your personal boundaries?

14. Did you notice that peer pressure played a part in your experience of this activity? If yes, how? What did you do about it?

15. If you had trouble getting through the tire inner tube, how did you feel about it? What did you think about yourself and your abilities? If you had negative thoughts about yourself and your abilities, what did you do about those thoughts? How could you have gone about changing any negative self-talk into more positive self-talk?

Sample Application-Processing Questions:

1. What are some other situations in which being optimistic or pessimistic about your chance of success would have an impact on the outcome? How can you apply what you learned about being optimistic or pessimistic to those situations?

2. How is your body image? How does your body image affect your attitudes and behaviors?

3. How do you usually handle being the center of attention?

4. What are some situations in your life in which you might have to do some things (like holding hands) that you don't want to do? How do you handle those situations? What did you learn in this activity that might make it easier for you to handle those situations?

5. When you have to talk in front of a group, how do you decide what to say? What impact does the setting have on what you decide to say?

6. What are some ways you are unique? What are some other situations in which you notice your own uniqueness? How can you celebrate that uniqueness?

7. What are some other situations in which you notice you have things in common with others? What kind of things do you have in common with others in those situations?

8. What are some other situations in which you might have to deal with peer pressure? How do you usually handle those situations? How can you apply what you might have learned in this activity about handling peer pressure to those situations?

9. What are some other situations in which you might need to ask for help? How do you usually handle those situations? How can you apply what you might have learned in this activity about asking for help in those situations?

10. What are some other situations in which you might have to trust others? How do you usually handle those situations? How can you apply what you might have learned in this activity about trusting others in those situations?

11. When you are in situations in which you are afraid you will fail, how do you usually react? What kinds of things do you usually tell yourself about yourself and your abilities?

12. How can you cultivate your ability to recognize negative self-talk? How can you get better at replacing negative self-talk with positive self-talk?

Safety Concerns:

1. Make sure the valve is cut out of the tire inner tube or that it is tied off in such a way that the valve can not scratch anyone.

2. In addition, you should be aware of the size of group members and any issues regarding body image. Even though you may know that the bicycle tire inner tube will stretch to fit anyone, some participants (especially if they are self-conscious) may feel anxious about doing this activity in front of others. We (at least Don and Jeff) often participate and go first, showing that the tire will fit over big guys and modeling a way to move through the tube without raising clothing in immodest ways.

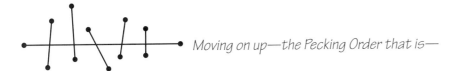

Moving on up—the Pecking Order that is—

Name of Activity: Pecking Order

Type of Activity: *Icebreaker; Deinhibitizer*

Grade Level: *First grade and up—as long as they can master Rock, Paper, Scissors*

Size of Group: *8 to 200 (no kidding—works with 200)*

Goal 2: Increase Self-Awareness and Self-Acceptance

Objectives:

   2A.   Explore personal attitudes and values
   2B.   Identify and acknowledge personal positive traits, talents, and accomplishments
   2C.   Develop ability to recognize negative self-talk
   2D.   Develop skills in replacing negative self-talk with positive self-talk
   2F.   Develop positive attitudes toward self
   2H.   Identify personal and social roles

Goal 6: Enhance Positive Attitudes and Skills Related to Learning

Objectives:

   6A.   Develop feeling of competence and confidence as a learner
   6B.   Take pride in accomplishments
   6C.   Accept mistakes as part of the learning process
   6D.   Apply time management and task management strategies
   6E.   Recognize that effort and persistence enhance learning
   6F.   Demonstrate dependability and initiative
   6H.   Develop critical-thinking skills

Materials: None

Preparation: None

How to Play:

1.   This is a game of progression based on challenging another participant to play Rock, Paper, Scissors. (Note: in case it has been a while: Paper covers Rock, Scissors cut Paper, and Rock breaks Scissors.)
2.   Participants progress (by winning a hand of Rock, Paper, Scissors) from an egg, to a chicken, to a hawk, to a pterodactyl.
3.   All participants begin as eggs. To symbolize eggs, participants should crouch near the ground to make themselves egg-shaped.
4.   Eggs can challenge other eggs to Rock, Paper, Scissors. The winner progresses to become a chicken while the loser remains an egg.
5.   Chickens should bend their arms at the elbows and make clucking noises (i.e., like a chicken).
6.   Chickens can challenge other chickens to Rock, Paper, Scissors. The winner progresses to a hawk, while the loser goes back to being an egg (e.g., crouching near the ground and looking for other eggs to challenge).
7.   Hawks should spread their arms out wide and straight as if they were soaring. (High-pitched screeching can also be encouraged depending on the space you are using—pretty funny.)
8.   Hawks can challenge other hawks to Rock, Paper, Scissors. The winner progresses to a pterodactyl, while the loser goes back to being an egg (e.g., crouching near the ground and looking for other eggs to challenge).
9.   Pterodactyls should raise their arms up high and do their best to look like the top of the pecking order.

10. Pterodactyls can challenge anyone (that's right—anyone!) to Rock, Paper, Scissors. If pterodactyls challenge (or are challenged by—yes, they can also be challenged) an egg, chicken, or hawk, and if the pterodactyl loses, the challenger progresses to the next level (i.e., egg to chicken, chicken to hawk, hawk to pterodactyl), but the pterodactyl does not regress to egg.
11. If the pterodactyl challenges another pterodactyl to Rock, Paper, Scissors, the winner stays a pterodactyl while the loser becomes an egg.

Variations:

It's not really a variation, but it is fun for you (the leader) to play. If you can get to the pterodactyl stage, you can wander around helping participants (especially those who are a little slow like our coauthor Don…) to move up from egg to another level. Note that if you're a pterodactyl, this comes at no real risk to you. We often tell participants, "I'm going to be a Rock," just to make sure they decide to be Paper so that they can progress to the next level.

Sample Personalization-Processing Questions:

1. What was your reaction when the leader first explained the rules?
2. If you were confused, what did you do to make sure you understood the rules?
3. How did you keep the rules of the game straight?
4. How did you feel when you had to go back to being an egg? How did you handle that experience?
5. How did the level you were at when you had to go back to being an egg affect how you reacted?
6. How did you feel when you got to go to the next level? What did you do to express those feelings?
7. How did your strengths (assets) serve you during this activity?
8. When you made a mistake and had to go back to being an egg, what did you tell yourself about yourself or your abilities? How did you notice if you were indulging in negative self-talk? How did you go about replacing negative self-talk with positive self-talk?
9. What did you learn from your mistakes?

Sample Application-Processing Questions:

1. What do you usually do to get clarity in situations in which you are confused by the directions for a task? How can you apply what you learned in this activity to those situations?
2. How do you feel about situations in which there are certain roles with more power than other roles? How do you handle it when you have a low-level role? How do you handle it when you have a high-level role?
3. Describe a time in which you felt successful in mastering a difficult task. How did you feel about your accomplishment? How did your feelings in that situation resemble your feelings in this activity?
4. Describe a time in which felt unsuccessful in mastering a difficult task. How did you feel about your lack of accomplishment? How did your feelings in that situation resemble your feelings in this activity?
5. What did you learn about yourself in this activity that could help in situations in which you feel successful? What about in situations in which you feel unsuccessful?
6. How do you usually react in situations in which your status is regularly challenged? How can effort, persistence, dependability, and initiative have an impact on your experience of this kind of situation?
7. Why is it important to keep trying even when things are difficult or you feel discouraged?
8. How can you be a good sport when your success means someone else's failure? Why is that important?

Safety Concerns: None

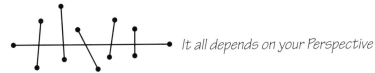 *It all depends on your Perspective*

Name of Activity: Perspectives

Type of Activity: Challenge/Initiative

Grade Level: Seventh grade and up

Size of Group: 15 to 30

Goal 1: Improve Communication and Relationship Skills

Objectives:

1D.   Express ideas clearly and constructively
1G.   Develop skills for making and maintaining relationships
1H.   Recognize and deal with peer pressure
1I.   Use communication skills to resolve conflict
1L.   Develop skills for effectively participating in groups

Goal 6: Enhance Positive Attitudes and Skills Related to Learning

Objectives:

6A.   Develop feeling of competence and confidence as a learner
6B.   Take pride in accomplishments
6C.   Accept mistakes as part of the learning process
6D.   Apply time management and task management strategies
6E.   Recognize that effort and persistence enhance learning
6F.   Demonstrate dependability and initiative
6G.   Develop the ability to share knowledge
6H.   Develop critical-thinking skills

Materials: The children's book Zoom *by Istvan Banyai (1995; available through Amazon.com, and relatively cheap)*

Note. The book *Zoom* is a wordless picture book that creates the effect of a camera lens zooming out. For example, the first illustration shows a girl playing with wooden farm pieces, the next illustration reveals the girl on a cover of a magazine, the next illustration shows the same (now smaller) magazine being held by a boy on a cruise ship. As the illustrations unfold, you see that the cruise ship is actually a poster on a bus. In this way, each page of the book is connected to the one immediately before and after it with the previous page appearing in smaller form on each subsequent page. The final picture shows a view of the earth from space.

Preparation: Remove the pages of the book Zoom *so each page can be distributed to a different participant. We have actually had our loose pages laminated for protection.*

How to Play:

1.   Give each participant a picture. That is, take as many pages of the book as there are participants (if 15 participants, then take the first 15 pages of the story), and randomly hand them out to the group participants.
2.   Have participants look at their pictures, but not show them to anyone else in the group.
3.   The goal is for the group to line up the pages in the correct sequential order of the story, as told by the pictures they are holding. In deciding this order, participants can use only verbal descriptions. So participants can look at their own pictures and try to describe them to other participants, but cannot show their pictures or look at others' pictures.
4.   When the group thinks everyone is in the correct spot, everyone can proceed to place his or her picture on the floor.
5.   Watch the fun as you see how the story unfolds—including any mistakes in the order.

Variations:

You may use the book *Re-zoom* by Istvan Banyai (1998) instead.

Sample Personalization-Processing Questions:

1. Did everyone feel heard as the group worked on solving the problem? If you didn't feel heard, what was that like for you? If you had wanted to be heard by the other members of the group, what could you have done differently to make sure that you were heard?
2. Did you communicate your ideas effectively? If so, how did you go about doing this? If not, what prevented you from doing this?
3. What process did the members of the group use to determine how to arrange the pictures? What were some things that would have made this process easier?
4. What were some of the ways that group members cooperated with one another to accomplish this task? How did cooperation help?
5. How did you decide whether to cooperate or not? How did your attitudes about cooperation influence what happened in the group? What about the attitudes of other group members?
6. If you disagreed with other members of the group about the order of the pictures, how did you express this disagreement? What were some more constructive, respectful ways to express disagreement?
7. Were you willing to consider the ideas of others? How could you have increased your willingness to consider other perspectives? How would this have been helpful if you had been willing to do it?
8. When members of the group disagreed on the order of the pictures, did you perceive this disagreement as a conflict? If the disagreement escalated into a conflict, how did you feel about the conflict? What did you do about your feelings? How did the group members resolve the conflict? What did you contribute to resolving the conflict? What would have been some other ways to do this?
9. What was your part in escalating the disagreement into a conflict? Was there something you could have done to prevent the disagreement from escalating into a conflict?
10. In what ways did peer pressure affect the process? How was the peer pressure communicated/exerted? How did the members of your group handle the peer pressure? How did you react to the peer pressure? Did you exert peer pressure on others during this process?
11. If the group made a mistake and arranged the pictures incorrectly, how did you feel about this mistake? How did you deal with your feelings? What did you communicate to the rest of the group when mistakes happened?
12. What did you learn from making a mistake that helped you in the rest of the process of this activity?
13. How did you feel when the group got the arrangement of the pictures right? How did you communicate those feelings to the rest of the group?
14. In what ways were effort and persistence important in this activity? Dependability and initiative? The ability to share knowledge? Critical-thinking skills? Time management skills?

Sample Application-Processing Questions:

1. How do you go about solving problems that are similar to the challenge presented in this activity? Which of the methods for problem solving used by the members of your group would be useful in other situations in your life? How can you use them in these situations?
2. Which of the methods for managing stress used by you or the members of your group could be helpful in other situations in your life? How can you apply them?
3. What are some other situations or relationships in which it might be important for you to be heard? How can you go about making sure that you are heard in those situations?
4. How can you apply some of the methods that you learned/practiced in this activity for communicating your ideas clearly?
5. How can you apply what you learned about learning from mistakes in other situations? Dealing with peer pressure?
6. How can you enhance your critical-thinking skills?
7. What are some other situations or relationships that would be improved if you were more respectful of the perspectives of others? What can you learn from listening to other people's perspectives? Why is it useful to listen to other people's perspectives?

8. What are some other situations in which you will need to exert effort and persistence in order to learn something? How can you apply what you learned in this activity to enhance your effort and persistence?
9. What are some other situations in which being dependable and showing initiative are important? How can you be more dependable and show more initiative in those situations?
10. What are some other situations in which you feel competent and confident as a learner? How can you increase these feelings of competence and confidence as a learner?
11. What are some ways that peer pressure can be positive? What are some ways peer pressure can be negative?

Safety Concerns: None

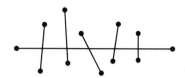

What are the Jewels of your school? Family? Community?
How do we nurture and protect these jewels?

Name of Activity: Protect the Jewels

Type of Activity: *Challenge/Initiative*

Grade Level: *Fifth grade and up*

Size of Group: *8 to 25*

Goal 1: Improve Communication and Relationship Skills

Objectives:

1D.   Express ideas clearly and constructively
1J.   Recognize the need for help and develop the ability to ask for it
1K.   Recognize and verbalize needs and wishes
1L.   Develop skills for effectively participating in groups

Goal 2: Increase Self-Awareness and Self-Acceptance

Objective:

2A.   Explore personal attitudes and values

Goal 3: Develop and Apply Problem-Solving and Decision-Making Skills

Objectives:

3A.   Set personal goals
3B.   Identify problems
3C.   Demonstrate understanding of steps for solving problems and making decisions (gather information; explore alternatives and consequences; plan and take action)
3D.   Evaluate decisions
3E.   Manage change and transitions in everyday life
3H.   Demonstrate effective coping skills for dealing with problems
3J.   Develop ability to identify alternative methods for solving problems and achieving goals

Materials: Handkerchief, soft ball, or sack/bag of some kind (e.g., mesh bag, plastic bag) to represent the jewels and a rope or some other boundary (e.g., masking tape)

Preparation: To play this game you need a circular (or at least some closed geometric shape) boundary. For instance, we often place a rope or a long piece of tape to create a circle approximately 10 to 15 feet in diameter. The area within the boundary needs to be large enough for group members to be able to place themselves around the perimeter with plenty of room between them.

How to Play:

1.   The handkerchief, ball, or bag represents the jewels or good stuff that one participant must try to protect from capture by other players. This Protector may not touch the jewels, but may stand or hover over them. (We often require all participants to stay on their knees in this activity.)
2.   The Protector positions him- or herself over or near the jewels, inside the perimeter, and everyone else forms a circle on their knees around the perimeter.
3.   When the activity begins, the players around the perimeter move in together to try to get the jewels safely out of the inner circle without being tagged by the Protector.
4.   If, while trying to get the jewels, a player is tagged by the Protector, he or she must return to the perimeter and come in again before again attempting to steal the jewels.

5. If a player successfully snags the jewels, and gets them out of the circle without being tagged by the Protector, that person becomes the Protector.
6. This game is cooperative in that players working together will be more successful. This may be discovered by the players themselves or can be subtly encouraged by the leader, depending on the group.[1]

Variations:

1. After playing a few rounds with just one Protector, add another Protector so you have two or three people in the middle protecting the jewels. Isn't it interesting how two people trying to protect the jewels or good stuff are more successful?
2. When players get tagged, they freeze in place and become obstacles to other players as they try to steal the jewels.
3. You can use the following metaphor in setting up the activity: After setting up the basic rules of the game, ask the participants, "What are the jewels of the school/community/family? What are the things you really like about the school/community/family that you want to protect and nurture?" You can even have students write these things down on 3 by 5 cards and put them in a small stuff sack. The stuff sack can become the jewels being guarded. After everyone identifies one characteristic, ask the participants, "What is something that could ruin one of the characteristics mentioned?" Answers might include not taking time, negativity, being mean, not caring, etc. Then, as participants crawl up to take the jewels, they can whisper whatever they think might rob the group of the good stuff. For example, a participant might whisper, "Here comes negativity, here comes negativity."
4. If you are playing the activity with more than one Protector guarding the jewels, you can identify what groups these additional Protectors might represent, such as teachers, students, administrators, parents, etc.

Sample Personalization-Processing Questions:

1. How did you decide who was going to be the Protector?
2. Did everyone feel heard in the process of choosing the Protector?
3. Were there people who wanted to be the Protector but didn't get chosen? If you were one of these people, how did it feel to not be chosen? What do you think you could have done differently to increase your chances of having what you wanted?
4. If you were a Protector, how did that feel? What was fun about being Protector? What was challenging about it?
5. If you were a Protector, what was your strategy for protecting the jewels? How did you figure out which strategy would be most effective? How did you decide if a strategy was not effective? How did you go about developing an alternative strategy if your strategy wasn't effective?
6. If you were a Protector and were successful in protecting the jewels, how did you feel about your success? If you were a Protector and someone stole the jewels, how did that feel? What did you tell yourself about your abilities if this happened?
7. If you were trying to steal the jewels, how did it feel when you met your goal and got the jewels? If you were not successful, how did you feel about that? What did you tell yourself about your abilities if this happened?
8. How did the people trying to steal the jewels interact with one another? Were you cooperating or competing?
9. How did the people who were trying to steal the jewels decide which strategy would be most effective? How did you decide if a strategy was not effective? How did you go about developing an alternative strategy if your strategy wasn't effective?
10. During the process of coming up with a strategy, what was the best way to get your ideas heard?
11. How did the transition between being a person who was trying to steal the jewels to being the Protector go?
12. How did it feel to go from being a Protector to being a person who was trying to steal the jewels?
13. How was the experience different when there was more than one Protector?

[1]*Note.* Adapted from Fluegelman, A. (1976). *The new games book.* San Francisco, CA: New Games Foundation.

14. If there was more than one Protector, how did they work together to make sure they were successful in protecting the jewels?
15. Was it easier or harder to protect the jewels with more people for the job?
16. How was this experience different when the people who were trying to steal the jewels froze in place when they were tagged, rather than going back out to the perimeter and starting over?
17. If the group used the metaphor of describing the jewels, what were the jewels? How did you decide what they were? Did your ideas get included?
18. Do you think it made the Protector more determined to protect the jewels when he or she knew exactly what was being protected?
19. How was it to be something that could rob the group of the good stuff?

Sample Application-Processing Questions:
1. How do you decide what is important to protect?
2. How do you go about protecting whatever is important to protect?
3. Describe a time when you have threatened something that was important to someone else. How did this come about? Looking back at the experience, how do you feel about what happened?
4. Is it easier to protect something that is important to you if you have other people to help you or do you prefer to work alone?
5. In these situations, how do you decide on the best strategy for protecting what is important?
6. If you are using a strategy to solve a problem, how do you decide whether that strategy is working?
7. If you decide a strategy is not working, how do you go about generating alternatives?
8. How do you usually handle transitions from one role to another? How could you apply what you learned in this activity about handing transitions to those situations?
9. Have you ever been in a relationship in which you felt as if you had to protect the other person? How was that experience for you? What strategies did you use? How did you decide whether the other person needed protecting in a particular situation?
10. Have you ever been in a relationship in which someone else was protecting you? How was that experience for you? Do you think you really needed protection?
11. How do you decide whether you need help? How do you go about asking for help?
12. What are some other situations in which cooperation is the best way to go about reaching your goal? What could you apply from today's experience in those situations?

Safety Concerns:
1. Play on a soft, even surface (i.e., grass). A gym floor will work, but is harder on a person's knees.
2. Make sure the Protector does not swing wildly in attempt to tag as many people as possible in a short time.

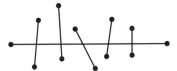

Name of Activity: Silver Lining

Type of Activity: *Icebreaker*

Grade Level: *Third grade and up*

Size of Group: *3 to 99 or more as long as you can have subgroups of 3 (It will actually work with any odd number of folks in each subgroup, but we think it is more fun with just 3.)*

Goal 1: Improve Communication and Relationship Skills

Objectives:

1D. Express ideas clearly and constructively
1G. Develop skills for making and maintaining relationships
1L. Develop skills for effectively participating in groups

Goal 2: Increase Self-Awareness and Self-Acceptance

Objectives:

2A. Explore personal attitudes and values
2C. Develop ability to recognize negative self-talk
2D. Develop skills in replacing negative self-talk with positive self-talk
2F. Develop positive attitudes toward self

Goal 3: Develop and Apply Problem-Solving and Decision-Making Skills

Objectives:

3E. Manage change and transitions in everyday life
3F. Apply decision-making skills to resolve conflicts
3H. Demonstrate effective coping skills for dealing with problems
3J. Develop ability to identify alternative methods for solving problems and achieving goals

Materials: None

Preparation: Divide the larger group into subgroups of three (or five or seven—really, whatever works with your numbers, but each subgroup needs to have an odd number of members).

How to Play:

1. Have each subgroup sit in a circle. In each group, ask for a volunteer to start a story.
2. Tell the group that they are going to practice a new skill, called *reframing*, in which they will learn to look for the silver lining in every cloud.
3. Ask the person who is going to start to think of something unfortunate that could happen to a person or group. They should tell the rest of their subgroup (in just one or two sentences, nothing too long-winded) what happened, starting their story with the word *unfortunately*. (For example, "Unfortunately, when the class went on their picnic, it began to rain.")
4. Going clockwise around the circle, the next person finds something constructive or fortunate that could also be a part of the story. Ask that he or she begin the next part of the story with *fortunately*. (For example, "Fortunately, they all brought umbrellas.")
5. The next person in the circle continues the story, but finds something unfortunate about the circumstances and begins the next part of the story with *unfortunately*. (For example, "Unfortunately, Luke's umbrella broke.")
6. The story continues around the circle, alternating fortunate and unfortunate circumstances until the story comes to a natural conclusion (or you tell them that time is up), ending on a positive,

note with something fortunate. (For example, "Fortunately, Luke had a crush on Carol, whose umbrella was still working." "Unfortunately, it was a small umbrella." "Fortunately, Carol also liked Luke, so being close together was fine with both of them." Etcetera, etcetera, etcetera.[1]

Sample Personalization-Processing Questions:

1. Which position was most comfortable for you—fortunately or unfortunately? What was comfortable about that position? What was uncomfortable about the other position?
2. What did you like about each of the positions? What did you dislike about each of the positions?
3. How did you feel about the story your group told? How did you feel about your contribution to the story? How did you express those feelings to your group?
4. How did it feel to be the center of attention when you were telling your part of the story?
5. How did you decide what to contribute to the story?
6. How did your contributions to the story reflect your personal attitudes and values?
7. How did you feel when the next person in the telling basically took the story in the opposite direction from the part you had just told?
8. Why was listening important in this activity? What did you do to make sure you were being a good listener?
9. How did you feel if the story went in a direction you did not feel comfortable with? What did you do to try to get the story back on a track with which you could feel comfortable?
10. If conflict occurred in your story, how did your group deal with it?
11. How did you feel about the constant transitions dictated by this activity? How did you deal with those transitions?

Sample Application-Processing Questions:

1. Are you usually a fortunately or an unfortunately person? In what ways?
2. What are some situations in which you would tend to be an unfortunately person? What are some situations in which you would tend to be a fortunately person? What changes for you in these different situations?
3. What did you learn from this activity about recognizing times when you are using negative self-talk? What can you learn from this activity about replacing negative self-talk with positive self-talk?
4. What are some situations or relationships in your life in which the circumstances tend to be negative? How do you usually handle these situations? How can you apply what you learned in this activity about finding the silver lining to those situations?
5. What are some situations or relationships in which you tend to be negative? How do you usually handle these situations? How can you apply what you learned in this activity about finding the silver lining to those situations?
6. What are some situations or relationships in which the other people involved tend to be negative? How do you usually handle these situations? How can you apply what you learned in this activity about finding the silver lining to those situations?
7. What are some situations or relationships in which you or others tend to be unrealistically optimistic and may need a reality check? How do you usually handle these situations? How can you apply what you learned in this activity about looking for the downside to those situations?
8. What are some other situations in which you are the center of attention? How do you feel about those situations? How do you handle being the center of attention?
9. Is it easier for you to tell a story to a small group (of, say, two other people) or to a bigger group? What do you think are the factors that influence your level of comfort?
10. When you have to tell a story in front of a group, how do you decide what to say? What impact does the setting or the audience have on what you decide to say?
11. What are some qualities that make a good storyteller? Which of those qualities do you possess?
12. What are some ways that what you have to say is unique? What are some other situations in which you notice your own uniqueness? How can you celebrate that uniqueness?

---

[1]*Note.* Adapted from Beaudion, M., & Walden, S. (1998). *Working with groups to enhance relationships.* Duluth, MN: Whole Person Associates.

13. What are some other situations in which you might have to deal with peer pressure? How do you usually handle those situations? How can you apply what you learned in this activity about handling peer pressure to those situations?

14. How can you apply what you learned about handling situations in which you disagree with the direction in which an experience is going to other situations?

15. What are some other situations or relationships in which it is important that you listen to others? What makes it important to listen to others in those situations or relationships?

Safety Concerns: As long as everybody keeps the gestures under control as they tell the story, you should have no problems. Right around the middle-school or junior-high age we begin to encourage participants to keep their stories in the G to PG range—

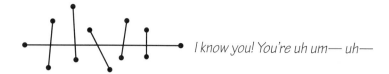
I know you! You're uh um— uh—

Name of Activity: Slide Show

Type of Activity: Icebreaker

Grade Level: First grade and up

Size of Group: 6 to 30

Goal 3: Develop and Apply Problem-Solving and Decision-Making Skills

Objectives:

3E.   Manage change and transitions in everyday life
3G.   Apply decision-making skills in life situations
3H.   Demonstrate effective coping skills for dealing with problems
3I.   Recognize when peer pressure is influencing decision making
3J.   Develop ability to identify alternative methods for solving problems and achieving goals

Goal 6: Enhance Positive Attitudes and Skills Related to Learning

Objectives:

6A.   Develop feeling of competence and confidence as a learner
6B.   Take pride in accomplishments
6C.   Accept mistakes as part of the learning process
6D.   Apply time management and task management strategies
6E.   Recognize that effort and persistence enhance learning
6F.   Demonstrate dependability and initiative
6G.   Develop the ability to share knowledge
6H.   Develop critical-thinking skills

Materials: Sheet, table cloth, curtain, or tarp that participants can't see through and can serve as a partition

Preparation: If you don't have a coleader, you will need to choose a helper who is about the same height as you are to hold the partition during the activity.

How to Play:

1.   This is a name and recognition game testing participants' speed and accuracy (i.e., how quickly can they recognize and correctly say the name of another participant).
2.   Divide the group into two roughly equal teams.
3.   Stand between the two newly formed teams and, along with your helper, hold up one end of the partition so that it is hanging lengthwise and opposing teams can hide behind it.
4.   Each team sends one member forward so that he or she is crouching or standing (depending upon how tall you and your helper are—and how tall the participants are) near the partition and facing the team on the other side.
5.   At this point, each team has sent one representative forward to stand very near the partition. The rest of the team is also hidden behind the partition so they cannot be seen by the other team. In this way, each team has a member forward, and neither team knows which member the other team has put forward.
6.   At this point, you and your helper, holding the ends of the partition count 1-2-3 and then drop the partition so that the two forward team members can suddenly see each other.
7.   The first forward member to correctly say the name of the other forward member wins.
8.   The loser joins the winning team, and the partition is raised again for another round.

9. Before each round of sending a team member forward, the team can strategize about who will go forward (e.g., "I'll bet that they think that we think that they think we'll put _____ forward").

10. The game is over when there is only one person left on a team (Gee, only one person left on that team—wonder who will be standing there when the partition drops) or, obviously, when you declare a winner.

Sample Personalization-Processing Questions:

1. How did your team decide whose name to call out?

2. How did the members of your team decide if a strategy was working? What did team members do if they decided a strategy wasn't working?

3. How did you feel when your team made a mistake and got a guess wrong? How did you express those feelings? What did you tell yourself about yourself and/or your abilities when you guessed incorrectly?

4. How did you feel when your team won? How did you express those feelings to the group? What did you tell yourself about yourself and/or your abilities when your team guessed correctly?

5. If you were pretty certain about whose name to call, did you try to influence the opinions of others in the group? If yes, what persuasive techniques did you use? Were there more effective ways for you to share your knowledge?

6. If other people expressed certainty about whose name to call, how did this affect your decision-making process? Did anyone try to persuade you to agree with their opinion?

7. Did these interactions feel like peer pressure? If yes, what part of the interactions felt like peer pressure? How did you cope with it?

8. How did you feel when your team lost, and you were the one who had to join the other team? What was this transition like for you? If the transition was difficult for you, what would have made it easier?

9. Were you correct more often or incorrect more often? How did you define whether you were successful at this activity? If you were successful, how did you feel about that? If you were unsuccessful, how did you feel about that?

10. How did you apply the learning from earlier turns as the game progressed?

11. How important was it for you to listen to the reasoning of other group members in the process of deciding whose name to call? Did their opinions affect your formation of your own opinion?

12. Did some of the interactions between group members feel like conflict to you? If yes, how did you handle the conflict? What were some ways you could have handled the conflict more effectively?

13. How did you apply your critical-thinking skills in this activity? What were some ways you could have used your critical-thinking skills more effectively?

14. What did you do to contribute to the success of the group?

Sample Application-Processing Questions:

1. As you were playing the game, did it feel really important that you call out the correct name? Was it really important that you did this? What do you think about the fact that it seemed important at the time, but might not have really been important?

2. What are some times in school when you get worried about something that might not really be important but you think it is at the time? At home?

3. What strategies can you use to determine whether something is really important? What are some ways you can get better at deciding whether something is really important?

4. What are other situations or relationships in your life in which others might try to influence your decisions? How can you apply what you learned in this activity in these situations?

5. What is your usual method of making decisions? How could you use what you learned in this activity to enhance your decision making?

6. Which of the methods for problem solving or decision making used by the members of this group would be useful in other situations in your life? How can you use them in these situations?

7. What are some other situations or relationships in which it might be useful for you to listen to others? How do you go about deciding whether to let yourself be influenced by listening to others?

8. How can you apply some of the methods of resolving conflicts that you learned/practiced in this activity in other situations?

9. How do you deal with situations in which you disagree with what the other members of a group decide? How can you apply what you learned in this activity to those situations?
10. What did you learn about your critical-thinking skills that you can apply to other situations in your life?
11. What are some situations in your life in which it is important to share your knowledge with others? How do you feel when you get to share your knowledge with others?
12. How can you apply some of the methods that you learned/practiced in this activity for dealing with peer pressure in other situations?
13. What are other situations or relationships in your life in which you need to make decisions about whether you are successful? How can you apply what you learned in this activity in these situations?
14. When you judge your performance as not being successful, how does this affect you? What do you tell yourself about yourself and/or your ability in those situations? What are some more positive ways for you to think about yourself and/or your abilities when you are not successful?

Safety Concerns: None

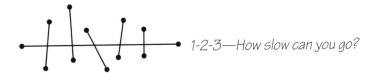 *1-2-3—How slow can you go?*

Name of Activity: Slow Motion Tag

Type of Activity: Icebreaker

Grade Level: Third grade and up

Size of Group: 8 to 40

Goal 2: Increase Self-Awareness and Self-Acceptance

Objectives:

2C.   Develop ability to recognize negative self-talk
2D.   Develop skills in replacing negative self-talk with positive self-talk
2E.   Appreciate own uniqueness
2F.   Develop positive attitudes toward self
2G.   Recognize personal boundaries, rights, and privacy needs
2H.   Identify personal and social roles

Goal 5: Demonstrate Consistently Responsible Behavior

Objectives:

5A.   Acknowledge personal responsibilities
5B.   Recognize whether behavior is appropriate and responsible
5C.   Act in an appropriate and responsible manner
5D.   Develop coping skills for dealing with stress
5E.   Understand the need for self-discipline and self-control and how to exercise them

Materials: None

Preparation: None, other than to designate a boundary or prescribed area

How to Play:

1. Have the group scatter in a prescribed area. The more people you have in the group, the larger the area needed. Ideally, the area would be just large enough that participants can spread out in the area and not touch anyone else. It is also helpful, and helps the game move more quickly, if participants are not too far apart.
2. Explain that this is a game of tag and that, in this game, everyone is It. The object is to tag others before they tag you. The catch in the game is that it is played in slow motion.
3. Participants are only allowed to move one step at a time. The rhythm of the game is for the leader to count "1—2—3—Move," and everyone to take one step when the leader says "Move." From this new position, participants try to avoid being tagged by others while trying to tag others.
4. When a participant is tagged, he or she simply exits the game. Tagged participants can gather around the perimeter and help the leader count, saying in unison with you "1—2—3—Move."

Variations:

You might try a moveable perimeter (like a rope or string). As the group shrinks in number, you can decrease the size of the perimeter, making it a little smaller and the game a little more exciting!

Sample Personalization-Processing Questions:

1. How was this game of tag different for you than other games of tag?
2. In this game of tag, there isn't a clear role distinction between the taggee and the tagger. How was it to have everyone be It?

3. Did you worry more about avoiding being tagged or tagging others? What do you think made that particular activity the most important thing for you?

4. How did you feel about someone else controlling your movement? How was it for you to have to move really slowly?

5. Were there times when you were telling yourself negative things about your ability to tag others? Your ability to move slowly? What kinds of things were you telling yourself?

6. How could you have changed this negative self-talk to more positive self-talk? What kinds of positive things could you tell yourself?

7. How did the way you went about this game differ from the way everybody else in the group went about the game?

8. How did you feel when the group stopped moving and someone was really close to you? How did that affect your sense of your personal boundaries?

9. What were your responsibilities to the group in this activity? How did you decide what your responsibilities were?

10. Did you honor those responsibilities in playing this activity? If yes, what kinds of things did you do that you felt were responsible? How did you make sure your behavior was responsible? If no, what kinds of things did you do that you felt were not responsible? What kept you from being responsible during this activity?

11. How could you tell whether other people perceived your behaviors as responsible? What kinds of feedback did you get from others (people in the group, the leader) about whether you were being responsible during this activity? How did you react when you got this kind of feedback?

12. What about this activity made it important to exercise self-discipline and self-control?

13. What did you find stressful in this activity? What strategies did you use to cope with this stress?

Sample Application-Processing Questions:

1. In relationships with friends, romantic partners (depending on the age—probably you don't want to include that part of the question with first and second graders, though times are a-changing), and family members, do you like to have a clear distinction between the pursuer or the pursued? How do you deal with it when there isn't that clear distinction?

2. Which role do you like best, pursuer or pursued? What do you like about that role? How often do you play the other role? What is uncomfortable for you about that role?

3. Are there other roles you play in your relationships (besides pursuer or pursued)? What are they? How often do you play these roles? How comfortable are you in each of these roles?

4. How do you handle it when you are in situations or relationships in which the roles are not clearly defined?

5. What are some other situations or relationships in which you might be telling yourself negative things about yourself or your abilities? How do you feel in these situations or relationships?

6. What are some strategies you have used for shifting your self-talk in a more positive direction?

7. What could you learn from this game that you could apply in situations in which it would be important to recognize and maintain your personal boundaries, rights, and privacy needs?

8. What are some situations in your life in which it feels as if others are in control of what you do and/or how you do it? How do you handle those situations?

9. What are some situations or relationships in your life in which you feel that it is really important to act in a responsible manner? How do you handle these situations or relationships?

10. What are some times when you do not act as responsibly as you think you should? What do you think keeps you from being responsible in those situations? How could you handle those situations differently in the future?

11. How do you feel when you get feedback that you are not acting in a responsible manner? How do you react to this feedback? How is your reaction affected by who it is that is giving the feedback?

12. How do you handle situations in which friends or family members are not acting responsibly? What kinds of feedback do you usually give in these situations? How do you handle situations in which acquaintances or strangers are not acting responsibly? What kinds of feedback do you usually give in these situations?

13. In what kinds of situations in your life do you feel the same kind of stress you felt during this activity? How can you apply what you learned about how you handle stress in this activity to those other situations?
14. What are some other situations in your life in which it is important to exercise self-control and self-discipline? How can you apply what you learned during this activity about your ability to exercise self-control and self-discipline to these situations?

Safety Concerns: Because participants are "frozen" in between steps, and sometimes these frozen poses are not that stable, we like to play on grass or some other soft surface.

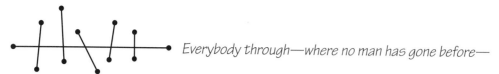

Everybody through—where no man has gone before—

Name of Activity: Star Gate

Type of Activity: Challenge/Initiative

Grade Level: First grade and up

Size of Group: 5 to 25 (more time with more people)

Goal 1: Improve Communication and Relationship Skills

Objectives:

1A.   Demonstrate understanding of and apply basic communication skills (e.g., recognizing nonverbal cues, delivering "I" messages)
1B.   Express feelings clearly and constructively
1C.   Recognize and accept the feelings of others
1D.   Express ideas clearly and constructively
1F.   Demonstrate willingness to trust others
1G.   Develop skills for making and maintaining relationships
1H.   Recognize and deal with peer pressure
1I.   Use communication skills to resolve conflict
1J.   Recognize the need for help and develop the ability to ask for it
1K.   Recognize and verbalize needs and wishes
1L.   Develop skills for effectively participating in groups

Goal 3: Develop and Apply Problem-Solving and Decision-Making Skills

Objectives:

3A.   Set personal goals
3B.   Identify problems
3C.   Demonstrate understanding of steps for solving problems and making decisions (gather information; explore alternatives and consequences; plan and take action)
3D.   Evaluate decisions
3G.   Apply decision-making skills in life situations
3H.   Demonstrate effective coping skills for dealing with problems
3I.   Recognize when peer pressure is influencing decision making
3J.   Develop ability to identify alternative methods for solving problems and achieving goals

Goal 4: Increase Understanding and Valuing of Diversity
(if you have a participant with a physical disability or you assign a disability to one or more participants; see Variations)

Objectives:

4A.   Recognize and appreciate individual differences
4D.   Acknowledge and appreciate similarities and differences across cultures and/or groups of people who have physical or learning differences
4E.   Recognize how stereotypes can affect interpersonal relationships and attitudes toward others

Goal 5: Demonstrate Consistently Responsible Behavior

Objectives:

5D.   Develop coping skills for dealing with stress
5E.   Understand the need for self-discipline and self-control and how to exercise them

Goal 6: Enhance Positive Attitudes and Skills Related to Learning

Objectives:

6B. Take pride in accomplishments
6C. Accept mistakes as part of the learning process
6D. Apply time management and task management strategies
6E. Recognize that effort and persistence enhance learning
6F. Demonstrate dependability and initiative
6G. Develop the ability to share knowledge
6H. Develop critical-thinking skills

Materials: Deflated bicycle inner tube (25 to 27 inches preferable)

Preparation: None

How to Play:

1. Have participants hold hands and stand in a circle (or a rough equivalent of a circle for those circle-challenged groups).
2. Have two members of the circle let go of one another's hands and grasp opposite sides of the inner tube. In this way the circle will be still be complete, but two folks will be holding on to the inner tube rather than each other's hands.
3. Instruct participants that the goal of the activity is for the entire group to pass through the inner tube that the two participants are holding. Note that the group must continue to hold hands and that the two designated participants must continue to hold the inner tube.
4. After a quick moment or two of raised eyebrows and possible confusion, it is likely to dawn on participants that the those on the opposite side of the circle can move toward the inner tube and make an effort to pass through the tire. It may also become clear that those holding the tire can help dramatically in facilitating participants' movement through the tire.
5. The activity ends with an inverted circle and a nice sense of accomplishment!

Variations:

1. This activity works well even if you have a person with a physical disability (e.g., is in a wheelchair). In fact, we like this dynamic so much, occasionally we assign a disability to one or more participant (e.g., take away sight, the use of arms). With this variation, a whole new set of processing issues can come up (see Goal 4).
2. As in Pass the Tire (p. 139), you can include two or more inner tubes in this activity. The circle can pass through one of the inner tubes, then pass through the other(s). This may make the activity a little longer (though once participants have figured out how to pass through the first tire, subsequent tires are usually easy for the group to navigate).
3. One variation we like is that the entire group must pass through the tube(s) but only the participants holding the tube in their hands can touch the tube. You can have the group keep trying until they pass through with no touches or have them try the activity with as few touches as possible. If you use the latter variation, you can also have groups set a goal for the number of touches—or keep trying until they can do it with no touches.

Sample Personalization-Processing Questions:

1. What was your initial reaction when the leader described the activity?
2. What did you think about the likelihood of getting the whole group through the inner tube? If you were pessimistic about the chances of getting the whole group through the tube, how did that affect your chances of getting through it? If you were optimistic about the chances of the whole group getting through the tube, how did that affect your chances of getting through it?
3. How might people's images of their bodies affect their reaction to this activity? How did your body image affect your reaction to this activity?
4. How did you feel about holding hands with the other people in the group? If you didn't want to hold hands, how did you handle it?
5. What about this activity required you to trust others? How was that experience for you?

6. How did you decide if you needed help getting through the inner tube? If you had to ask for help from others to get through the tube, how did you feel about that? How did you go about asking for help? How could you have gotten more comfortable with asking for help?

7. How did it feel to be the center of attention, going through the inner tube? How did you express those feelings to the group? If it was hard for you to be the center of attention during this process, what was hard about it? Was there something you or some other member of the group could have done to make this easier for you?

8. How did being the center of attention affect your stress level? How did you deal with it if you felt stressed out?

9. How did the members of the group handle the problem of getting everyone through the inner tube? Did they just start going or did they strategize first? How did you feel about the way the group went about this task?

10. If the group did strategize, what did you contribute to the process?

11. If you wanted to share knowledge or information with the rest of the group, how did you go about making sure you were heard?

12. How did the members of the group determine whether the strategy for getting everyone through the tube was working? If it wasn't working, how did the members of the group generate alternative strategies?

13. Did you have any stereotypes that affected your perspective on certain people going through the inner tube? What was the impact of you holding those stereotypes?

14. Did you notice that peer pressure played a part in your experience of this activity? If yes, how? What did you do about it?

15. Why was listening important in this activity? How did you do as a listener in this activity? How could you have improved your listening?

16. What role did trust play in this activity? What could you and the other members of the group have done to enhance trust in the group?

17. Why was cooperation important in this activity? What were some of the ways that the members of the group cooperated with one another to accomplish this task? How did cooperation help?

18. What role did you play in this process (leader? follower? observer?)? Did the group need someone to be the leader to be able to get everyone through? If so, how did you work out who was going to lead and who was going to follow? Did the roles change during the course of the activity? How?

19. If group members disagreed on strategies for getting everyone through the inner tube, did you define that disagreement as conflict? If yes, how did you feel about the conflict? What did you do about your feelings? How did the members of the group resolve the conflict? What would have been some other ways to do this?

20. How did you feel about it when the group was successful in getting through the inner tube?

21. On a 1 to 10 scale, how stressful was this activity for you? What made it stressful? Where did you feel the stress in your body? What could you have done to make the activity less stressful for you?

22. Were there any instances in which peer pressure affected the group members during this process? What impact did peer pressure have on you? What did you do to cope with peer pressure?

23. If you had someone in your group with a physical challenge, how did the group handle that?

24. What were some ways that the group was able to convey respect about differences among people?

Sample Application-Processing Questions:

1. In what other situations or relationships in your life does it feels as though you must work with other people to make something happen? What resources/strategies do you have to help you deal with these situations?

2. What part does cooperation play in these situations or relationships? How do you elicit cooperation and help?

3. What are some other situations in which stereotypes might influence your interactions with others? How can you make sure that you reduce the possibility of this happening in the future?

4. How do you usually go about solving problems? Which of the methods for problem solving used by the members of the group would be useful in other situations in your life? How can you use them in these situations?

5. What are some other situations in which you might need to ask for help? How can you go about recognizing that you need help and asking for it?

6. What are some other situations or relationships in which it might be important for you to be heard? How can you go about making sure that you are heard in those situations?

7. What are some other situations or relationships in which it might be important for you to be a good listener? How can you go about making sure that you are using effective listening skills in those situations?

8. What are some other situations or relationships in which you need to use your conflict resolution skills? How can you apply some of the methods that you learned/practiced in this activity for appropriately resolving conflicts in these situations?

9. What could you learn from this activity that you could apply in situations in which it would be important to share information with others? Use critical-thinking skills?

10. What are some other situations in your life in which trusting others is important? How can you apply what you learned about trusting others in this activity to those other situations?

11. In what kind of situation in your life do you decide to be a leader? How do you go about leading? In what kind of situation in your life do you decide to be a follower? How do you go about following? In what kind of situation in your life do you decide to be an observer? How do you go about observing?

12. What are some other situations in which being optimistic or pessimistic about your chance of success would have an impact on the outcome? How can you apply what you learned about being optimistic or pessimistic to those situations?

13. How is your body image? How does your body image affect your attitudes and behaviors?

14. How do you usually handle being the center of attention?

15. What are some situations in your life that you might have to do some things (like holding hands) that you don't want to do? How do you handle those situations? What did you learn in this activity that might make it easier for you to handle those situations?

16. What are some other situations in which you might have to deal with peer pressure? How do you usually handle those situations? How can you apply what you might have learned in this activity about handling peer pressure to those situations?

17. What are some other situations in which you might have to trust others? How do you usually handle those situations? How can you apply what you might have learned in this activity about trusting others to those situations?

Safety Concerns: It may be important to monitor how participants are passing through the inner tube (e.g., some groups decide to lift people off the ground).

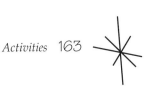

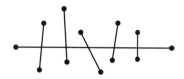

This game is one that can get pretty wild, so think about the level of aggression and impulse control in your group and don't play with members who will want to cream each other—and may the Force be with you.

Name of Activity: Star Wars Dodge Ball

Type of Activity: *Deinhibitizer; Challenge/Initiative*

Grade Level: *First grade and up*

Size of Group: *10 to 100*

Goal 3: Develop and Apply Problem-Solving and Decision-Making Skills

Objectives:

3A. Set personal goals
3B. Identify problems
3C. Demonstrate understanding of steps for solving problems and making decisions (gather information; explore alternatives and consequences; plan and take action)
3D. Evaluate decisions
3E. Manage change and transitions in everyday life
3H. Demonstrate effective coping skills for dealing with problems
3J. Develop ability to identify alternative methods for solving problems and achieving goals

Goal 5: Demonstrate Consistently Responsible Behavior

Objectives:

5A. Acknowledge personal responsibilities
5B. Recognize whether behavior is appropriate and responsible
5C. Act in an appropriate and responsible manner
5D. Develop coping skills for dealing with stress
5E. Understand the need for self-discipline and self-control and how to exercise them
5G. Demonstrate respect for alternate perspectives

Goal 6: Enhance Positive Attitudes and Skills Related to Learning

Objectives:

6A. Develop feeling of competence and confidence as a learner
6B. Take pride in accomplishments
6C. Accept mistakes as part of the learning process
6E. Recognize that effort and persistence enhance learning
6F. Demonstrate dependability and initiative
6G. Develop the ability to share knowledge
6H. Develop critical-thinking skills

Materials: Open space, two sticks that can be used as reanimation wands, something to use as a divider between the two teams (can be masking tape or a rope) and balls. (We use sock balls, which are balls made by taking old, clean socks and rolling them inward on themselves so that the toe of the sock is all that is left, but you can also use any soft ball that can be thrown without hurting whoever it hits.) The number of balls you need will vary, depending on how big your group is and how active your members are. The more the merrier, though, regardless of the group.

Preparation: Put your room divider down the middle of your space, with the balls distributed along the divider.

How to Play:

1. Divide the group into two teams. We just arbitrarily divide them into teams, rather than letting them pick teams. (Several of us still have PTSD from always being the last person picked for teams in elementary school.)
2. Appoint a Luke Skywalker or Princess Leia (or other Jedi Master) for each team. This person is now the team's reanimation expert, wielding the reanimation wand for that team. (Note: You can let the team choose a person, you can appoint a person you think needs more status in the group, or you can let someone volunteer for the position.)
3. Explain that they will be playing dodge ball with several new rules: The object of the game is to freeze all of the people on the other team. Tell them, "The way you can freeze folks is to hit them with a ball. When you are hit with a ball, the way to get unfrozen is to attract the attention of your team's Luke Skywalker or Princess Leia and have them touch you with the reanimation wand. The only person who can use the wand is the designated expert.
4. Let them take a few minutes to develop a strategy that they believe will work; and then let them know when you give the starting signal they can run up, get the balls, and start throwing at the other team. Then (and this is the really important part of these directions), get out of the way (because otherwise, you might be frozen, which we certainly wouldn't want) and give them the starting signal.
5. When all of the members of one team are frozen, the other team is declared the winner!

Variations:

1. You can tell the group that the reanimation expert is the most important person on each team before you start, or you can let them figure that out the hard way—by being wiped out by the other team when their Luke or Princess gets hit and they have no chance to be reanimated, which signs the death warrant for the team.
2. You can add other rules, such as, "If a person on the other team catches a ball you have thrown, then you are frozen."
3. One thing we like to do is to play several rounds, with a strategy session in between—with maybe a little nudge or two from us to suggest that it is REALLY important to protect the only person who can unfreeze them. We might also have them develop better strategies for asking for help.

Sample Personalization-Processing Questions:

1. What was fun for you about this activity?
2. What was hard (or frustrating) for you about this activity?
3. Who was the most important person on your team? What was so important about that person?
4. How did your team go about protecting that person?
5. When you had a chance to strategize, did the members of your team actually develop a team strategy for protecting your most important person? If no, how did that work out for your team? If yes, how did you decide what would be the best way/a better way to protect that person?
6. How did your team members decide whether your strategy for protecting your most important person was working? What did the members of your team do about it if you decided the strategy wasn't working as well as you wanted it to work?
7. Did your team have a team strategy for getting the other team frozen? If no, how did that work for you? If yes, how did you decide on that strategy? What did the members of your team do about it if you decided the strategy wasn't working as well as you wanted it to work?
8. Did you have an individual strategy for accomplishing what you wanted to accomplish during this activity? If yes, how did you decide on that strategy? What did you do about it if you decided the strategy wasn't working as well as you wanted it to work?
9. How did you feel when you got frozen? How did you handle it when you got frozen?
10. How did you get help when you were frozen? How did you feel about having to ask for help?
11. When you got hit, were you always honest about getting hit/being frozen? How did you decide whether to choose to be honest or not? How did you feel when you chose to be honest? How did you feel when you chose not to be honest?

12. How did you feel when you observed someone else choosing not to be honest about getting frozen? How did you handle this situation? What were some other ways you could have handled this situation?

13. If you saw several different people choosing not to be honest, did you have different reactions depending on your relationship with each person? How did your reaction change? What were the factors that influenced your reaction?

14. What did you learn from the first or second round of the game that you applied to later rounds?

15. What was your level of stress during this activity? How did it change as time passed? What strategies did you use to cope with the stress involved in this activity?

16. When members of the group disagreed on strategies for getting the other team frozen or for protecting the important person, how did you feel about the disagreement? What did you do about your feelings? How did the group members resolve the conflict? What would have been some other ways to do this?

17. In what ways did peer pressure affect the members of your team? How did you handle the peer pressure?

18. What did you contribute to the effort of your team?

19. If you were feeling discouraged during this activity, how did you deal with that? What did you find discouraging? What did you tell yourself to increase your motivation? If other members of your team were feeling discouraged, how did you interact with them about their discouragement?

20. How did you feel about it if your team won by freezing all the members of the other team? How did you feel if your team was the one with all the members frozen? How did you communicate those feelings to the rest of your team or the other team?

21. What were your responsibilities to your team in this activity? What were your responsibilities to the entire group in this activity? How did you decide what your responsibilities were?

22. Did you honor those responsibilities in playing this activity? If yes, what kinds of things did you do that you felt were responsible? How did you make sure your behavior was responsible? If no, what kinds of things did you do that you felt were not responsible? What kept you from being more responsible?

23. How did you decide whether your team was successful? How did you decide whether you, personally, were successful?

24. For the Princess/Luke/Jedi Master: How did you feel about being the most important person in your group? Did your feelings about being the most important person on your team change over the process of the activity? What was stressful for you about the job of reanimation expert? What was fun about the job? How did you feel about being protected? How did you feel when the protection didn't work well? How did you ask for better protection? How did you cope with all those people clambering for help? How did you feel when you got frozen?

Sample Application-Processing Questions:

1. How do you define success in other situations in your life? How can you apply what you learned in this activity about yourself and the way you think and feel about success to other situations in your life?

2. What are other situations or relationships in your life in which it feels as though you must dodge missiles at the same time you are throwing missiles? What resources do you have to help you deal with these situations?

3. What are some other situations in your life in which you must have cooperation and help (work as a team) to be successful? How do you deal with these situations? How do you elicit cooperation and help?

4. How do you go about solving problems that are similar to incoming and outgoing missiles? To having someone in your life who needs to be protected? Which of the methods for problem solving used by the members of your team would be useful in other situations in your life? How can you use them in these situations?

5. Which of the methods for managing stress you tried in this activity can be helpful in other situations in your life? How can you use them?

6. What are some other situations in which you might need to ask for help? How can you go about recognizing that you need help and asking for it? How can you enhance your ability to accept help when it is offered?

7. How can you apply what you learned during this activity about dealing with mistakes in other situations? Dealing with peer pressure?
8. What did you learn about your critical-thinking skills that you can apply to other situations in your life?
9. What are situations in your life in which it is important to choose to be honest? How do you usually handle those situations? How do you decide whether to be honest in those situations?
10. What are some situations in your life in which you need to count on other people's honesty? How do you decide how you want to handle those situations in which someone is not honest?
11. What are some situations in which you believe it is acceptable not to be honest? Why is it all right to choose to be dishonest in those situations?
12. What are some situations in your life in which you feel responsible or take responsibility for others? How can you apply what you learned in this activity about being responsible or taking responsibility in these other situations?
13. What are some situations in which you might need protection? How can you recognize situations in which you need protection? How can you go about getting protection in those situations? How can you enhance your ability to accept protection when it is offered?
14. How do you decide what is really important to you in life? How can you go about making those really important things a priority for you?

Safety Concerns: Watch out for those balls. You can make rules that automatically freeze anyone who hits someone in the head if you think that is a way to keep folks safe.

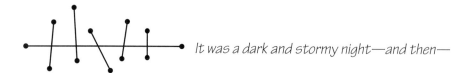 *It was a dark and stormy night—and then—*

Name of Activity: Stretching Story

Type of Activity: Icebreaker; Deinhibitizer

Grade Level: First grade and up

Size of Group: 1 to 20 (If there is just one participant, simply pass the story back and forth between the two of you—big fun as you get to determine where the plot goes next.)

Goal 1: Improve Communication and Relationship Skills

Objectives:

- 1A. Demonstrate understanding of and apply basic communication skills (e.g., recognizing nonverbal cues, delivering "I" messages)
- 1B. Express feelings clearly and constructively
- 1D. Express ideas clearly and constructively
- 1E. Listen actively to others
- 1G. Develop skills for making and maintaining relationships
- 1J. Recognize the need for help and develop the ability to ask for it
- 1L. Develop skills for effectively participating in groups

Goal 2: Increase Self-Awareness and Self-Acceptance

Objectives:

- 2A. Explore personal attitudes and values
- 2B. Identify and acknowledge personal positive traits, talents, and accomplishments
- 2C. Develop ability to recognize negative self-talk
- 2D. Develop skills in replacing negative self-talk with positive self-talk
- 2E. Appreciate own uniqueness
- 2F. Develop positive attitudes toward self
- 2G. Recognize personal boundaries, rights, and privacy needs
- 2H. Identify personal and social roles

Goal 4: Increase Understanding and Valuing of Diversity

Objectives:

- 4A. Recognize and appreciate individual differences
- 4B. Develop an understanding and appreciation of own culture
- 4C. Demonstrate respect for others as both individuals and members of different cultural groups
- 4D. Acknowledge and appreciate similarities and differences across cultures and/or groups of people who have physical or learning differences
- 4E. Recognize how stereotypes can affect interpersonal relationships and attitudes toward others

Materials: None

Preparation: None

How to Play:

1. In this activity, the group shares a story by having each group member tell a part. In addition, the storyteller acts out what is happening in the story, and the rest of the group mimics the storyteller's actions.

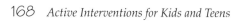

2. Begin by having the group form a circle and by explaining to the participants that they are going to take turns telling a story together, which they will act out as they go. Each person in the group who is doing the storytelling also decides how to act out that part of the story, while the participants doing the listening copy the actions of the talker.
3. After every few lines of the story, the storytelling (and acting out) role is passed to the next person in the circle.
4. We usually begin the story making ourselves the narrator so we can act out whatever we are doing in the story (e.g., "I was out for a walk one evening when. . ."). You may need to remind the group to walk with you as you walk in place describing your evening stroll. After a few lines, you pass the story to the participant next to you, using a transitional phrase such as "and then" that allows the participant to pick up the thread and continue the story.
5. The story is passed around the circle until it comes back to you, and you can wrap it up in a flourish.
6. By going first, you model how much of the story to tell (i.e., how long to talk). With a larger group, this can go on too long if each of your 15 group members takes 3 minutes (yawn!). If a particular participant is either hogging the story, or seems to have gotten lost in the plot and doesn't seem to know how to get out, we often interrupt by saying loudly "and then" to move it along to the next person.

Variations:

1. To more easily accomplish Goal 2, you can give a context for the story being about a particular person and his or her self-awareness and self-acceptance. For instance, you could say, "Let's tell a story about two friends, one very self-confident and the other full of self-doubt." or "Let's tell about the different groups of kids who go to a school—like some are the popular kids, some are trouble-makers, some are really smart."
2. To more easily accomplish Goal 4, you can set up the story to talk about a particular culture or group of people by starting the story with an request to tell the story about that particular culture or group of people (i.e., "Let's tell a story about some people who live in Africa" or "Let's tell a story about something that happened in the projects in New York City" or "Let's tell a story about a very small town and what happens there").

Sample Personalization-Processing Questions:

1. How did it feel to be the center of attention, telling the story?
2. What direction did you take the story? Did you talk about scary things, sad things, funny things, etc.? How did you decide where to take the story?
3. How did you decide whether to take the story in the same direction as the previous story tellers or in a new direction?
4. How were the things you added to the story different from what others added? What did you notice about how your uniqueness was reflected in the part you told?
5. How were the things you added to the story similar to the things that other people added? What did you notice having in common with others in the group?
6. How did your part of the story express your personal attitudes and values?
7. How did you feel when the person before you was telling his or her part of the story, making you the next person to talk? As that person talked, how did you prepare to tell your part of the story?
8. How did you feel when it was time to pass the story on to the next person?
9. How did peer pressure affect the direction of the story? How did you deal with that peer pressure?
10. How did your part of the story reflect your culture? How did your culture influence how you felt about talking?
11. Why was listening important in this activity? What did you do to make sure you were being a good listener?
12. How did you feel if the story went in a direction you did not feel comfortable with? What did you do to try to get the story back on a track about which you could feel comfortable?
13. If the group used Variation 1, what did the story tell about feeling good about yourself?
14. If the group used Variation 1, what did you learn from the story about recognizing when you are using negative self-talk? What did the story tell about replacing negative self-talk with positive self-talk?

15. If the group used Variation 2, what did you learn about the culture highlighted in the story? How did the story express respect for that culture? Were there ways in which the story illustrated similarities and differences among cultures?

16. If the group used Variation 2, were stereotypes part of the story? How did you feel about this? If you were uncomfortable with stereotypes that were played out in the story, what did you do about your discomfort? How could you have more constructively given feedback to the group about stereotypes?

Sample Application-Processing Questions:

1. What are some other situations in which you are the center of attention? How do you feel about those situations? How do you handle being the center of attention?

2. When you have to tell a story in front of a group, how do you decide what to say? What impact does the setting have on what you decide to say?

3. What are some qualities that make a good storyteller? Which of those qualities do you possess?

4. What are some ways that what you have to say is unique? What are some other situations in which you notice your own uniqueness? How can you celebrate that uniqueness?

5. What are some other situations in which you might have to deal with peer pressure? How do you usually handle those situations? How can you apply what you learned in this activity about handling peer pressure to those situations?

6. How can you apply what you learned about handling situations in which you disagree with the direction in which an experience is going to other situations?

7. What ways does your culture influence your actions and relationships? How can you become more aware of how your culture affects your actions and relationships? How can you become more aware of how other people's cultures affect their actions and relationship? How can you be more respectful of other people's cultures?

8. How can you apply what you have learned today about your own culture and the cultures of others to reduce the number of stereotypes you hold and help you view other people in a more realistic and respectful way?

9. How do your personal attitudes and values have an impact on your relationships? How can what you learned in this activity about your personal attitudes and values help you in expressing your values and attitudes in more constructive ways?

10. What are some other situations or relationships in which it is important that you listen to others? What makes it important to listen to others in those situations or relationships?

11. What are some other situations in which you might notice people expressing stereotypes? How do you usually feel about those situations? How do you usually handle those situations? How can you apply what you might have learned in this activity to help you communicate more clearly and constructive to others about stereotypes?

Safety Concerns: None, unless it is a dangerous story.

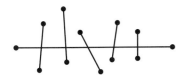

That's Stretching it a bit, don't you think?

Name of Activity: Stretching the Limit

Type of Activity: Challenge/Initiative

Grade Level: Third grade and up

Size of Group: 6 to 60, depending on how much space you have

Goal 1: Improve Communication and Relationship Skills

Objectives:

- 1A. Demonstrate understanding of and apply basic communication skills (e.g., recognizing nonverbal cues, delivering "I" messages)
- 1D. Express ideas clearly and constructively
- 1E. Listen actively to others
- 1H. Recognize and deal with peer pressure
- 1I. Use communication skills to resolve conflict
- 1K. Recognize and verbalize needs and wishes
- 1L. Develop skills for effectively participating in groups

Goal 2: Increase Self-Awareness and Self-Acceptance

Objectives:

- 2G. Recognize personal boundaries, rights, and privacy needs
- 2H. Identify personal and social roles

Goal 3: Develop and Apply Problem-Solving and Decision-Making Skills

Objectives:

- 3A. Set personal goals
- 3H. Demonstrate effective coping skills for dealing with problems
- 3I. Recognize when peer pressure is influencing decision making
- 3J. Develop ability to identify alternative methods for solving problems and achieving goals

Goal 5: Demonstrate Consistently Responsible Behavior

Objectives:

- 5A. Acknowledge personal responsibilities
- 5B. Recognize whether behavior is appropriate and responsible
- 5C. Act in an appropriate and responsible manner
- 5D. Develop coping skills for dealing with stress
- 5E. Understand the need for self-discipline and self-control and how to exercise them
- 5F. Apply time management skills
- 5G. Demonstrate respect for alternate perspectives

Materials: None

Preparation: No preparation is necessary, but some space is needed for this activity. The more people you have, the more space is needed.

How to Play:

1. The object of this activity is for the group to see how long a continuous line they can make using only their bodies and any spare equipment that they have on them such as belts, shoelaces, hats, extra clothes, etc.

2. Explain to the group that all participants and items must be connected and laid end to end to form the line.
3. Give the group a time limit to organize and create their line with a solid countdown at the end to assure no confusion as to when the line has to be completed.
4. If you have more than one group, have the groups compete against one another.
5. Once groups have completed their lines, leaders can verify the length and place an object to mark the accomplishment of the group.[1]

Variations:

Have each group set a goal and see if the group meets or exceeds this goal. After the activity, the group can process how the goal was set and the group process in completing the task. In many cases, the group will move far beyond their initial goal.

Sample Personalization-Processing Questions:

1. What process did the members of the group use to decide on a strategy for making their line?
2. What did you do to contribute to the success of the group? How do you feel about your contribution?
3. How did the members of the group decide on what their goal was? How did they evaluate whether this goal was achievable?
4. If there was more than one group, did you compare your goal to the goals of the other groups? Did you compare the length of your line to theirs? What were the effects of this comparison?
5. Did you feel heard as the group members worked on making the line? How did it feel when you were heard by other members of the group?
6. If you didn't feel heard, what was that like for you? If you had wanted to be heard by the other members of the group, what could you have done differently to make sure that you were heard?
7. Did you communicate your ideas effectively? If so, how did you go about doing this? If not, what prevented you from doing this?
8. What did you do in your role as a listener to make the process of making the line go more smoothly?
9. What were some of the ways that group members cooperated with one another to accomplish this task? How did cooperation help?
10. How did you decide whether to cooperate or not? How did your attitudes about cooperation influence what happened in the group? What about the attitudes of other group members?
11. What role did you have in the process of strategizing about making the line? In actually making the line? What roles did other group members play in the process of making the line? How did the group members work out who was going to lead and who was going to follow? Did the roles change during the course of the activity? How?
12. How did you feel about being physically close and/or touching one another as you made the line? If you felt uncomfortable with the physical closeness and/or touching one another during this activity, what did you do about it?
13. In what ways did peer pressure affect the process? How did you and/or the other members of your group handle the peer pressure?
14. If you met or exceeded your goal, how did that feel? If you failed to meet your goal, how did that feel?
15. How did you express your needs and wishes in this process? What did you do if your needs and wishes were not met?
16. What were your responsibilities to yourself in this activity? What were your responsibilities to the group? How did you decide what your responsibilities were?
17. Did you honor those responsibilities in playing this activity? Did you tend to pay more attention to your responsibilities to yourself or to your responsibilities to the group? What was that about? What kinds of things did you do that you felt were responsible? How did you make sure your behavior was responsible? What kinds of things did you do that you felt were not responsible? What kept you from being more responsible?
18. What was your level of stress during this activity? How did the time limit affect your stress level? What strategies did you use to cope with the stress involved in this activity?

[1] *Note.* Adapted from Cain, J., & Jolliff, B. (1998). *Teamwork and teamplay.* Dubuque, IA: Kendall Hunt.

Sample Application-Processing Questions:

1. How could you get more comfortable setting limits or boundaries around personal space or touch?
2. What are some other situations in your life in which you must have cooperation and help (work as a team) to be successful? How do you deal with these situations? How do you elicit cooperation and help?
3. How do you set goals for yourself? What did you learn from this activity about setting and meeting personal goals?
4. How did the role(s) you played in this group resemble your role(s) in your family? In other groups? How do the other roles taken by various group members resemble roles taken by the other people in your life? What is your comfort level with these various roles?
5. How do you go about solving problems that are similar to the situation in this activity? Which of the methods for problem solving used by the members of your group would be useful in other situations in your life? How can you use them in these situations?
6. Which of the methods for managing stress used by you or the members of your group could be helpful in other situations in your life? How can you use them?
7. What are some other situations in which you might need to ask for help? How can you go about recognizing that you need help and asking for it? What can you do that might enhance your ability to accept help?
8. What are some other situations or relationships in which it might be important for you to be heard? How can you go about making sure that you are heard in those situations?
9. What are some other situations in which you might need to tell others about your needs and/or wishes? How can you go about getting better at recognizing when you have needs and/or wishes? What are some ways you can go about asking for what you want and/or need?
10. How can you apply some of the methods for communicating about ideas, encouraging cooperation, solving problems, and/or appropriately resolving conflicts that you learned/practiced in this activity in other situations?
11. How can you apply what you learned about dealing with stress in other situations? Dealing with peer pressure?
12. What could you learn from this game that you could apply in situations in which it would be important to recognize and maintain your personal boundaries, rights, and privacy needs?
13. What are the rules (spoken or unspoken) about personal space and/or touching in your family? In your culture?
14. What are some other situations in your life in which being responsible is important? How can you apply what you learned in this activity about being responsible to those other situations?
15. What are some of your responsibilities to yourself? How can you pay more attention to your responsibilities to yourself?

Safety Concerns: None, although you may want to set parameters about what clothes can be taken off to stretch the limit.

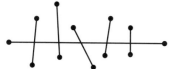 *Yes, we'd like to—But we're all tied up!*

Name of Activity: Tied Up in Knots

Type of Activity: *Deinhibitizer; Challenge/Initiative*

Grade Level: *Third grade and up*

Size of Group: *5 to 20*

Goal 1: Improve Communication and Relationship Skills

Objectives:

1A.   Demonstrate understanding of and apply basic communication skills (e.g., recognizing nonverbal cues, delivering "I" messages)
1B.   Express feelings clearly and constructively
1C.   Recognize and accept the feelings of others
1D.   Express ideas clearly and constructively
1E.   Listen actively to others
1F.   Demonstrate willingness to trust others
1G.   Develop skills for making and maintaining relationships
1H.   Recognize and deal with peer pressure
1I.   Use communication skills to resolve conflict
1J.   Recognize the need for help and develop the ability to ask for it
1K.   Recognize and verbalize needs and wishes
1L.   Develop skills for effectively participating in groups

Goal 2: Increase Self-Awareness and Self-Acceptance

Objectives:

2B.   Identify and acknowledge personal positive traits, talents, and accomplishments
2C.   Develop ability to recognize negative self-talk
2D.   Develop skills in replacing negative self-talk with positive self-talk
2G.   Recognize personal boundaries, rights, and privacy needs

Goal 3: Develop and Apply Problem-Solving and Decision-Making Skills

Objectives:

3A.   Set personal goals
3B.   Identify problems
3C.   Demonstrate understanding of steps for solving problems and making decisions (gather information; explore alternatives and consequences; plan and take action)
3D.   Evaluate decisions
3E.   Manage change and transitions in everyday life
3F.   Apply decision-making skills to resolve conflicts
3G.   Apply decision-making skills in life situations
3H.   Demonstrate effective coping skills for dealing with problems
3I.   Recognize when peer pressure is influencing decision making
3J.   Develop ability to identify alternative methods for solving problems and achieving goals

Goal 4: Increase Understanding and Valuing of Diversity

Objectives:

4A.   Recognize and appreciate individual differences
4B.   Develop an understanding and appreciation of own culture

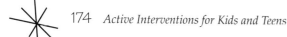

4C. Demonstrate respect for others as both individuals and members of different cultural groups

4D. Acknowledge and appreciate similarities and differences across cultures and/or groups of people who have physical or learning differences

4E. Recognize how stereotypes can affect interpersonal relationships and attitudes toward others

Goal 5: Demonstrate Consistently Responsible Behavior

Objectives:

5B. Recognize whether behavior is appropriate and responsible

5C. Act in an appropriate and responsible manner

5D. Develop coping skills for dealing with stress

5E. Understand the need for self-discipline and self-control and how to exercise them

5G. Demonstrate respect for alternate perspectives

Goal 6: Enhance Positive Attitudes and Skills Related to Learning

Objectives:

6A. Develop feeling of competence and confidence as a learner

6B. Take pride in accomplishments

6C. Accept mistakes as part of the learning process

6D. Apply time management and task management strategies

6E. Recognize that effort and persistence enhance learning

6F. Demonstrate dependability and initiative

6G. Develop the ability to share knowledge

6H. Develop critical-thinking skills

Materials: Rope long enough to accommodate all of the group participants holding on to the rope with both hands—with 3 to 4 feet between each participant (e.g., for 10 people—30 to 40 feet of rope)

Preparation: Tie several loose knots in the rope. (Note: The more knots the longer the activity will take.)

How to Play:

1. Lay out the rope (with knots tied in it) on the floor in front of the group.
2. Invite all of the participants to spread out and pick up the rope with two hands.
3. Instruct participants to grasp the rope such that there are no knots between any one participant's two hands.
4. Explain that once participants have grasped the rope with both hands, they are not to let go of the rope with either hand until the activity is complete.
5. Finally, explain that the group task is to, without letting go of the rope, untie all of the knots in the rope.
6. Sometimes we ask participants to stop midway through the activity and process/brainstorm how they could be more successful.

Variations:

1. Have the participants attempt the activity with a time limit (varies depending on the talent and stage of the group and the difficulty of the knots).
2. Have the participants set a time goal (e.g., "we can untie these knots in _____ minutes").

Sample Personalization-Processing Questions:

1. Did everyone feel heard as the group worked on solving the problem? If you didn't feel heard, what was that like for you? If you had wanted to be heard by the other members of the group, what could you have done differently to make sure that you were heard?
2. Did you communicate your ideas and feelings effectively? If so, how did you go about doing this? If not, what prevented you from doing this?
3. What process did the members of the group use to determine how to go about the untying?

4. What were some of the ways that group members cooperated with one another to accomplish this task? How did cooperation help?

5. How did you decide whether to cooperate or not? How did your attitudes about cooperation influence what happened in the group? What about the attitudes of other group members?

6. How could you tell whether you needed help from other group members? What did you do when you needed help? How did you ask for help when you recognized you needed it?

7. What roles did various group members play in the process of untying? How did the group members work out who was going to lead and who was going to follow? Did the roles change during the course of the activity? How?

8. How did you feel about being physically close as you untied the knots? How much personal space do you need? How is this different from the other people in the group and their personal space requirements?

9. What was your level of stress during this activity? How did it change as time passed? If you had a time limit, did this affect your stress level? What strategies did you use to cope with the stress involved in this activity?

10. When members of the group disagreed on strategies for untying the knots, how did you feel about the conflict? What did you do about your feelings? How did the group members resolve the conflict? What would have been some other ways to do this?

11. In what ways did peer pressure affect the process? How did the members of your group handle the peer pressure?

12. What personal positive traits and talents did you bring to this process and how did you use them to help in the untying?

13. How did you decide what methods to use in the untying? How did you decide whether the method you chose was working? If it wasn't working, how did you generate new ideas, and how did you decide which ones to use?

14. If the group made a mistake and made the knots worse, or you had a knot that the group could not untangle, how did you feel about that? How did you deal with your feelings? What did you tell yourself about your abilities? What did you tell yourself about the other members of the group? What did you communicate to the rest of the group when mistakes happened?

15. If you were feeling discouraged, how did you deal with that? What did you tell yourself to motivate yourself to continue? If other group members were feeling discouraged, how did you interact with them about their discouragement?

16. How did you feel about it when you got a knot untied? How did you communicate those feelings to the rest of the group?

17. What were your responsibilities to the group in this activity? How did you decide what your responsibilities were?

18. Did you honor those responsibilities in playing this activity? If yes, what kinds of things did you do that you felt were responsible? How did you make sure your behavior was responsible? If no, what kinds of things did you do that you felt were not responsible? What kept you from being responsible during this activity?

Sample Application-Processing Questions:

1. How did the knots in this activity resemble situations in your family? Your friendships? Other relationships?

2. How did the role you played in this group resemble your role in your family? In other groups? How do the other roles taken by various group members resemble roles taken by the other people in your life?

3. How do you go about solving problems that are similar to a collection of knots? Which of the methods for problem solving used by the members of your group could be useful in other situations in your life? How can you use them in these situations?

4. Which of the methods for managing stress that you or the members of your group used would be helpful in other situations in your life? How can you use them?

5. What are some other situations in which you might need to ask for help? How can you go about recognizing that you need help and asking for it?

6. What are some other situations or relationships in which it might be important for you to be heard? How can you go about making sure that you are heard in those situations?

7. How can you apply some of the methods for communicating about feelings and ideas, encouraging cooperation, solving problems, and/or appropriately resolving conflicts that you learned/practiced in this activity in other situations?

8. How can you apply what you learned about dealing with mistakes in other situations? Dealing with negative self-talk? Encouraging persistence and flexibility? Dealing with peer pressure? Dealing with stress? What could you learn from this game that you could apply in situations in which it would be important to recognize and maintain your personal boundaries, rights, and privacy needs?

9. What are the rules (spoken or unspoken) about personal space in your family? In your culture?

10. What are some other situations in which you have noticed differences in people's comfort levels about personal space? What were the differences that you noticed?

11. What have you noticed about different cultural groups and their rules about personal space?

12. If someone else has different rules than you do about personal space, how can you handle this in an appropriate and respectful way?

13. What did you learn about your critical-thinking skills that you can apply to other situations in your life?

14. What are some other situations in your life where you could notice and celebrate your own uniqueness? Your talents, abilities, contributions? Your successes?

Safety Concerns: None

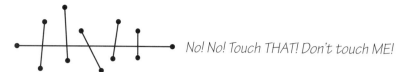 *No! No! Touch THAT! Don't touch ME!*

Name of Activity: Touch My Can

Type of Activity: *Trust; Challenge/Initiative*

Grade Level: *Third grade and up*

Size of Group: *8 to 40*

Goal 1: Improve Communication and Relationship Skills

Objectives:

1A. Demonstrate understanding of and apply basic communication skills (e.g., recognizing nonverbal cues, delivering "I" messages)
1B. Express feelings clearly and constructively
1C. Recognize and accept the feelings of others
1D. Express ideas clearly and constructively
1E. Listen actively to others
1F. Demonstrate willingness to trust others
1G. Develop skills for making and maintaining relationships
1J. Recognize the need for help and develop the ability to ask for it
1K. Recognize and verbalize needs and wishes
1L. Develop skills for effectively participating in groups

Goal 2: Increase Self-Awareness and Self-Acceptance

Objective:

2G. Recognize personal boundaries, rights, and privacy needs

Goal 3: Develop and Apply Problem-Solving and Decision-Making Skills

Objectives:

3A. Set personal goals
3B. Identify problems
3C. Demonstrate understanding of steps for solving problems and making decisions (gather information; explore alternatives and consequences; plan and take action)
3D. Evaluate decisions
3H. Demonstrate effective coping skills for dealing with problems
3J. Develop ability to identify alternative methods for solving problems and achieving goals

Goal 4: Increase Understanding and Valuing of Diversity

Objectives:

4A. Recognize and appreciate individual differences
4B. Develop an understanding and appreciation of own culture
4D. Acknowledge and appreciate similarities and differences across cultures and/or groups of people who have physical or learning differences

Goal 5: Demonstrate Consistently Responsible Behavior

Objectives:

5A. Acknowledge personal responsibilities
5B. Recognize whether behavior is appropriate and responsible

5C. Act in an appropriate and responsible manner

5D. Develop coping skills for dealing with stress

5E. Understand the need for self-discipline and self-control and how to exercise them

Materials: The only material required for the activity is something that the group can touch. We like to use an aluminum can (like a soft drink can) or bottle. However, you can use a rock, stapler, or any other object that you have handy and that you think will be funny. Note that the smaller the object, the harder the task.

Preparation: None

How to Play:

1. Explain to the group that the object of the activity is for every participant to touch (literally make continuous physical contact with) the can (or whatever object you've chosen) all at the same time.

2. Also explain that all participants must touch the can WITHOUT touching each other.

Variations:

1. Sometimes we ask the group to hold the position of all touching the can, while not touching each other, long enough to sing a song, give a cheer, etc.

2. For a more challenging variation, require the group to not come into contact with each other at any point in the activity (e.g., not just ending up touching the can and not touching each other, but completing the activity without touching each other at any time or they have to start again).

Sample Personalization-Processing Questions:

1. What was your reaction when you first heard the directions to this activity? How did you express your thoughts and feelings? Did your reaction change as the group discussed strategies? How?

2. What did you do to contribute to the success of the group? How did you feel about your contribution?

3. Did you feel heard as the group members worked on solving the problem? How did it feel when you were heard by other members of the group?

4. If you didn't feel heard, what was that like for you? If you had wanted to be heard by the other members of the group, what could you have done differently to make sure that you were heard?

5. Did you communicate your ideas and feelings effectively? If so, how did you go about doing this? If not, what prevented you from doing this?

6. What did you do in your role as a listener to make the process in this activity go more smoothly?

7. What role did trust play in this activity?

8. What process did the members of the group use to determine how to go about touching the can and not touching one another? How did the group members decide whether a strategy was working? If a strategy wasn't working, how did the group members deal with that? How did you go about developing an alternative strategy when something wasn't working?

9. What were some of the ways that group members cooperated with one another to accomplish this task? How did cooperation help?

10. How did you decide whether to cooperate or not? How did your attitudes about cooperation influence what happened in the group? What about the attitudes of other group members?

11. How could you tell whether you needed help from other group members? What did you do when you needed help? How did you ask for help when you recognized you needed it?

12. What roles did various group members play in the process of touching the can and not touching one another? How did the group members work out who was going to lead and who was going to follow? Did the roles change during the course of the activity? How?

13. How did you feel about being physically close at the same time you were avoiding touching one another? How much personal space do you need? How is this different from the other people in the group and their personal space requirements?

14. How did you decide if you needed or wanted something from the other members of the group? How did you go about asking for what you needed/wanted?

15. On a 1 to 10 scale (with 1 being no stress and 10 being a huge amount of stress), what was your level of stress during this activity? How did it change as time passed? If you had to sing a song while touching the can, how did this affect your stress level? If you had to start over if someone touched another person, how did this affect your stress level? What strategies did you use to cope with the stress involved in this activity?

16. Why did this activity require self-control and self-discipline? How did you do with that?

17. Was your group successful in your quest? How did you feel about your success or lack of success? How did you communicate those feelings to the rest of the group?

18. What were your responsibilities to the group in this activity? How did you decide what your responsibilities were?

19. Did you honor those responsibilities in playing this activity? If yes, what kinds of things did you do that you felt were responsible? How did you make sure your behavior was responsible? If no, what kinds of things did you do that you felt were not responsible? What kept you from being more responsible?

20. How was the way you approached this task different than the way the other people in the group approached it? How was the way you approached this task similar to the way the other people in the group approached it?

21. What are the messages in your culture about being different than other people? What are the messages in your culture about success?

22. If using Variation 2: How did it feel if someone touched someone else in the process and the whole group had to start over? How did it feel if you were that person? What did the various members of the group communicate to one another if this happened?

Sample Application-Processing Questions:

1. What are other situations or relationships in your life in which it feels as if you have to do something that seems impossible to do? What resources/strategies do you have to help you deal with these situations?

2. What are some other situations in your life in which you must have cooperation and help (work as a team) to be successful? How do you deal with these situations? How do you elicit cooperation and help?

3. How do you usually contribute to the success of a group process? What gifts do you bring to the world?

4. How did the role(s) you played in this group resemble your role(s) in your family? In other groups? How do the other roles taken by various group members resemble roles taken by the other people in your life? What is your comfort level with these various roles?

5. How do you go about solving problems that are similar to the situation in this activity? Which of the methods for problem solving used by the members of your group would be useful in other situations in your life? How can you use them in these situations?

6. Which of the methods for managing stress that you or the members of your group used could be helpful in other situations in your life? How can you use them?

7. What are some other situations in which you might need to ask for help? How can you go about recognizing that you need help and asking for it?

8. What are some other situations or relationships in which it might be important for you to be heard? How can you go about making sure that you are heard in those situations?

9. How can you apply some of the methods for communicating about feelings and ideas, encouraging cooperation, and/or appropriately resolving conflicts that you learned/practiced in this activity in other situations?

10. How can you apply what you learned about solving challenging problems?

11. What could you learn from this game that you could apply in situations in which it would be important to recognize and maintain your personal boundaries, rights, and privacy needs?

12. What are the rules (spoken or unspoken) about personal space and/or touching in your family? In your culture?

13. What are some other situations in which you have noticed differences in people's comfort levels about personal space and/or physical touch? What were the differences that you noticed? If someone else has different rules than you do about personal space, how can you handle this in an appropriate and respectful way?
14. What have you noticed about different cultural groups and their rules about personal space and/or physical touch?
15. What did you learn about your critical-thinking skills that you can apply to other situations in your life?
16. What are some other situations in your life in which acting responsibly is important? How can you apply what you learned in this activity about acting responsibly to those other situations?
17. What are some other situations in your life in which trusting others is important? How can you apply what you learned about trusting others in this activity to those other situations?
18. What are some other situations in your life in which communicating about your needs and/or wishes is important? How can you apply what you learned in this activity about communicating about your needs and/or wishes to those other situations?

Safety Concerns: Because participants sometimes get creative in body posture to avoid touching each other and still touch the can, we like to try and play on grass or some other soft surface.

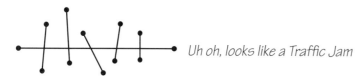
Uh oh, looks like a Traffic Jam

Name of Activity: Traffic Jam

Type of Activity: *Challenge/Initiative*

Grade Level: *Sixth grade and up (This activity can be frustrating for adult groups, is often easier for younger groups; there is probably a lesson there—)*

Size of Group: *8 to 20*

Goal 1: Improve Communication and Relationship Skills

Objectives:

1A.   Demonstrate understanding of and apply basic communication skills (e.g., recognizing nonverbal cues, delivering "I" messages)
1B.   Express feelings clearly and constructively
1C.   Recognize and accept the feelings of others
1D.   Express ideas clearly and constructively
1E.   Listen actively to others
1F.   Demonstrate willingness to trust others
1G.   Develop skills for making and maintaining relationships
1H.   Recognize and deal with peer pressure
1I.   Use communication skills to resolve conflict
1J.   Recognize the need for help and develop the ability to ask for it
1K.   Recognize and verbalize needs and wishes
1L.   Develop skills for effectively participating in groups

Goal 2: Increase Self-Awareness and Self-Acceptance

Objectives:

2C.   Develop ability to recognize negative self-talk
2D.   Develop skills in replacing negative self-talk with positive self-talk
2F.   Develop positive attitudes toward self
2G.   Recognize personal boundaries, rights, and privacy needs

Goal 3: Develop and Apply Problem-Solving and Decision-Making Skills

Objectives:

3A.   Set personal goals
3B.   Identify problems
3C.   Demonstrate understanding of steps for solving problems and making decisions (gather information; explore alternatives and consequences; plan and take action)
3D.   Evaluate decisions
3E.   Manage change and transitions in everyday life
3F.   Apply decision-making skills to resolve conflicts
3G.   Apply decision-making skills in life situations
3H.   Demonstrate effective coping skills for dealing with problems
3I.   Recognize when peer pressure is influencing decision making
3J.   Develop ability to identify alternative methods for solving problems and achieving goals

Goal 5: Demonstrate Consistently Responsible Behavior

Objectives:

5B.   Recognize whether behavior is appropriate and responsible

5C.   Act in an appropriate and responsible manner

5D.   Develop coping skills for dealing with stress

5E.   Understand the need for self-discipline and self-control and how to exercise them

5F.   Apply time management skills

Goal 6: Enhance Positive Attitudes and Skills Related to Learning

Objectives:

6A.   Develop feeling of competence and confidence as a learner

6B.   Take pride in accomplishments

6C.   Accept mistakes as part of the learning process

6D.   Apply time management and task management strategies

6E.   Recognize that effort and persistence enhance learning

6F.   Demonstrate dependability and initiative

6G.   Develop the ability to share knowledge

6H.   Develop critical-thinking skills

Materials: Enough markers (e.g., pieces of tape, rubber spots, place mats) for each person in the group to have one—plus one additional marker.

Preparation: Place the markers on the ground in either a straight or curved (half-moon shaped) line.

How to Play:

1.   Have each participant stand on a marker, leaving one marker in the middle free.

2.   Have the participants on each side of the open marker in the middle face the other participants on the other side.

3.   Instruct the participants that the goal of the activity is for the participants to change places with the participants on the other side of the empty marker following these rules:

   a.   Only one person can move at a time.

   b.   Participants can only move forward.

   c.   Participants can only move forward on to an empty mark directly in front of them or pass a single participant facing the opposite direction, moving around him or her on to an empty mark.

   d.   If the group gets stuck (e.g., no one can move and still comply with the rules because there are no appropriate empty spaces to move into, or the group realizes they've made a tragic error and are going to be stuck soon), they can step off the marks and line up again in their original order to try again.

Variations:

1.   After the group has been successful (figured it out), have them do it again as fast as they can. After they do it as fast as they can, have them set a goal for how fast they can do it.

2.   After the group has been successful, have the group complete the task in silence.

3.   Bring the activity out again at a later time, whether the group was successfully initially or not.

Note. This is a challenging puzzle to figure out. Groups often surprise us by getting it quickly or never getting it. True story: A group of aeronautical engineers tried repeatedly and couldn't complete the activity. Upon reflection, one commented, "Well, it's not like we're rocket scientists—" Which is exactly what they were.

Sample Personalization-Processing Questions:

1.   What did you feel/think about the group's chances for success when the leader first explained the rules? How did you express your thoughts and feelings? How did your initial attitude affect your approach to solving the problem?

2.   What did you do to contribute to the group solving the puzzle? How did you feel about your contribution?

3.   If your group didn't successfully solve the puzzle, how was that for you? How did you handle this failure? What did you tell yourself about yourself and your abilities related to this failure?

What did you tell yourself about the other group members related to this failure? How could you have dealt with this more constructively?

4. If your group successfully solved the puzzle, how was that for you? How did you handle this success? What did you tell yourself about yourself and your abilities related to this success? What did you tell yourself about the other group members related to this success? Was there some way you could have dealt with this more constructively?

5. If the group did solve the puzzle and the leader asked you to do it again, as quickly as you could, how did you feel about this?

6. How important was communication between you and the other members of the group in this activity?

7. Did you feel heard by the other members of the group as you worked to solve the puzzle? How did it feel when you were heard by the other group members?

8. If you didn't feel heard, what was that like for you? If you had wanted to be heard by your partner, what could you have done differently to make sure that you were heard?

9. Did you communicate your ideas and feelings effectively? Did you communicate your needs and wishes effectively? If so, how did you go about doing this? If not, what prevented you from doing this?

10. How did you do as a listener in this activity? How could you have improved your listening?

11. What role did trust play in this activity? What could you have done to enhance trust between the members of the group? What could other group members have done to enhance trust?

12. What process did you and the other members of the group use to determine how to go about solving the puzzle? How did you decide whether a strategy was working? If a strategy wasn't working, how did you deal with that? How did you go about developing an alternative strategy when something wasn't working?

13. What were some of the ways that members of the group cooperated with one another to accomplish this task? How did cooperation help?

14. How did you decide whether to cooperate or not? How did your attitudes about cooperation influence what happened among the members of the group?

15. How could you tell whether you needed more help from the other members of the group? What did you do when you needed more help? How did you ask for more help when you recognized you needed it?

16. What roles did each member of the group play in the process of solving the puzzle? Did one of you need to be the leader to have the group be successful? If so, how did you work out who was going to lead and who was going to follow? Did the roles change during the course of the activity? How?

17. If you and the other members of the group disagreed on strategies for solving the puzzle, how did you feel about the disagreement? What did you do about your feelings? Did the disagreement escalate into a conflict? How did you deal with the conflict? What would have been some other ways to do this?

18. If you were feeling discouraged and/or frustrated in this process, how did you deal with that? What did you tell yourself to motivate yourself to continue? If other members of the group were feeling discouraged, how did you interact with them about the discouragement?

19. What did you learn from failed attempts to solve the puzzle? How did you use that learning to perfect your strategies for solving the puzzle?

20. What were your responsibilities to the group in this activity? How did you decide what your responsibilities were?

21. Did you honor those responsibilities in playing this activity? If yes, what kinds of things did you do that you felt were responsible? How did you make sure your behavior was responsible? If no, what kinds of things did you do that you felt were not responsible? What kept you from being more responsible?

22. Were there times when you were telling yourself negative things about your ability to solve the puzzle? What kinds of things were you telling yourself?

23. How could you have changed this negative self-talk to more positive self-talk? What kinds of positive things could you tell yourself?

24. What part did effort and persistence play in whether you and the other members of the group were successful in solving the puzzle?

25. As you were working on solving the puzzle, did you compare your contribution to the process to the contribution of others? How did that comparison affect you and your efforts?
26. If you had more than one group working on solving this puzzle, did you look around and compare your group to other groups? How did that affect you and your efforts?

Sample Application-Processing Questions:

1. In what other situations or relationships in your life does it feel as though you must work with other people to make something happen? What resources/strategies do you have to help you deal with these situations?
2. What part does cooperation play in these situations or relationships? How do you elicit cooperation and help?
3. How did the role you had in the group resemble your role in your family? With friends? How flexible are you about roles?
4. How do you go about solving problems that are similar to the situation in this activity? Which of the methods for problem solving used by you and the members of the group would be useful in other situations in your life? How can you use them in these situations?
5. What are some other situations in which you might need to ask for help? How can you go about recognizing that you need help and asking for it? What are some other situations in which you might need to ask for what you want and/or need? How can you go about recognizing that you want and/or need something and asking for it?
6. What are some other situations or relationships in which it might be important for you to be heard? How can you go about making sure that you are heard in those situations?
7. What are some other situations or relationships in which it might be important for you to be a good listener? How can you go about making sure that you are using effective listening skills in those situations?
8. How can you apply some of the methods for communicating about feelings and ideas, encouraging cooperation, solving problems, and/or appropriately resolving conflicts that you learned/practiced in this activity in other situations?
9. How can you apply what you learned about dealing with negative self-talk?
10. What could you learn from this game that you could apply in situations in which it would be important to share information with others?
11. What did you learn about your critical-thinking skills that you can apply to other situations in your life?
12. What are some other situations in your life in which taking responsibility is important? How can you apply what you learned in this activity about taking responsibility to those other situations?
13. What are some other situations in your life in which trusting others is important? How can you apply what you learned in this activity about trusting others to those other situations?
14. What are some other situations in which you have felt like a success? How have you handled these situations? How can you apply what you learned in this activity to those situations?
15. What are some other situations in which you have felt like a failure? How have you handled these situations? How can you apply what you learned in this activity to those situations?
16. What are some other situations or relationships in which you compare yourself to others? What has the impact of those comparisons been on you and/or your relationships? How can you apply what you learned in this activity about comparing yourself to others to those situations or relationships?
17. How do you usually deal with frustration? How can you apply what you learned in this activity about handling frustration in those situations?

Safety Concerns: None except potentially strong frustration until they get it.

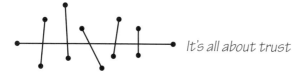
It's all about trust

Name of Activity: Trust Walk

Type of Activity: *Trust*

Grade Level: *First grade and up*

Size of Group: *2 to ??? (the sky's the limit— as long as safety isn't an issue)*

Goal 1: Improve Communication and Relationship Skills

Objectives:

- 1A.   Demonstrate understanding of and apply basic communication skills (e.g., recognizing nonverbal cues, delivering "I" messages)
- 1B.   Express feelings clearly and constructively
- 1C.   Recognize and accept the feelings of others
- 1D.   Express ideas clearly and constructively
- 1E.   Listen actively to others
- 1F.   Demonstrate willingness to trust others
- 1G.   Develop skills for making and maintaining relationships
- 1H.   Recognize and deal with peer pressure
- 1J.   Recognize the need for help and develop the ability to ask for it
- 1K.   Recognize and verbalize needs and wishes
- 1L.   Develop skills for effectively participating in groups

Goal 2: Increase Self-Awareness and Self-Acceptance

Objectives:

- 2A.   Explore personal attitudes and values
- 2B.   Identify and acknowledge personal positive traits, talents, and accomplishments
- 2C.   Develop ability to recognize negative self-talk
- 2D.   Develop skills in replacing negative self-talk with positive self-talk
- 2E.   Appreciate own uniqueness
- 2F.   Develop positive attitudes toward self
- 2G.   Recognize personal boundaries, rights, and privacy needs
- 2H.   Identify personal and social roles

Goal 5: Demonstrate Consistently Responsible Behavior

Objectives:

- 5A.   Acknowledge personal responsibilities
- 5B.   Recognize whether behavior is appropriate and responsible
- 5C.   Act in an appropriate and responsible manner
- 5D.   Develop coping skills for dealing with stress
- 5E.   Understand the need for self-discipline and self-control and how to exercise them

Materials: You may choose to use blindfolds—in which case, we use rolled bandanas (easy to launder—and come in lots of fun colors).

Preparation: Thinking about a safe path to have participants walk—with just enough of a challenge.

How to Play:

1.   Have participants find (or, if appropriate, assign) partners.
2.   Have the pair decide who is going first.

3. Explain that in the activity one of the partners will be sightless (either blindfolded or with eyes closed).
4. Explain that the sighted partner (without the blindfold or with eyes open) needs to make every effort to keep his or her partner safe, assist him or her in following you (the leader), and keep silent until the walk is over.
5. Lead the group (moving in pairs) in a walk. Gauge the walk based on your assessment of the group and your ability to spot for safety. For instance, you might take one group out a set of double doors—but not another group (because you might not be assured that the sighted partners will be mindful enough to keep their partners from being smacked by the door). If you have a coleader, you might lead a particular group down an incline because your coleader can monitor safety of the pairs as they move down the incline—while you are still leading the group.
6. After the first part of the walk is over, ask participants to switch roles.
7. Repeat steps 3 through 5.

Variations:

1. Have the sighted partner remain silent during the walk.
2. Have the sighted partner remain silent for part of the walk and provide a stream of encouraging feedback for the other part of the walk.

Sample Personalization-Processing Questions:

1. What was it like to be the sighted partner? How did you feel about leading your partner? Did your feelings change during the course of the activity? If yes, what changed for you?
2. What was it like to be the blind partner? How did you feel about being led by your partner? Did your feelings change during the course of the activity? If yes, what changed for you?
3. Which role did you like better? What did you like about that role? What didn't you like about the other role?
4. How did you feel about being out of control when you were being led?
5. How did you feel about being responsible when you were leading?
6. When you were being led, how difficult was it for you to let your partner know what you needed?
7. When you switched roles, did your partner have different needs than you? How did he or she communicate this?
8. When you were sighted, what did you do to help your partner feel more comfortable and safe? Were your efforts successful? How did your partner communicate about this? Which of the methods you used worked? Which ones didn't work?
9. When you were blind, what did your partner do to help you feel more comfortable and safe? Which methods worked? Which ones didn't work? How did you communicate with your partner about this?
10. In listening to the members of the group discuss this, were there patterns in the feelings and needs of the partner who was blind? Of the partners who were sighted?
11. This activity is called Trust Walk. How was trust involved?
12. In what ways did you trust your partner? In what ways were you mistrustful of your partner? How did your level of trust affect your interactions?
13. What were your responsibilities to your partner in this activity? What were your responsibilities to the group in this activity? How did you decide what your responsibilities were?
14. Did you honor those responsibilities during this activity? If yes, what kinds of things did you do that you felt were responsible? How did you make sure your behavior was responsible? If no, what kinds of things did you do that you felt were not responsible? What kept you from being responsible during this activity?
15. How could you tell whether other people perceived your behaviors as responsible? What kinds of feedback did you get from others (your partner, other people in the group, the leader) about whether you were being responsible during this activity? How did you react when you got this kind of feedback?
16. Did you feel that your partner was responsible during this activity? What kind of feedback did you give your partner about his or her being responsible (or not) during this activity?
17. How did your partner's ability to act in a responsible way affect your ability to trust him or her?

18. What about this activity made it important to exercise self-discipline and self-control?
19. On a 1 to 10 scale, how stressful was this activity for you? What made it stressful? Where did you feel the stress in your body? What strategies did you use to cope with this stress? What would have made it less stressful for you?
20. What did you learn about yourself during this activity? What did you learn about your partner?

Sample Application-Processing Questions:

1. In other situations in your life, how do you decide what role (leader or follower) you are going to play?
2. In what other situations or relationships in your life does it feels as though you are trying to do something blind? How do these situations affect you? How do you feel in these situations? What strategies do you use to cope with these situations? How can you apply what you learned in this activity to these situations?
3. What are some other situations in which you might need to depend on someone else for help? How can you go about recognizing that you need help and asking for it?
4. What are some other situations in which someone else needs your help? How can you be most helpful in these situations?
5. What are some other situations in which you might need to ask for what you need? How can determine what you need? How can you get more comfortable asking for what you need?
6. What are some other situations or relationships in which it might be important for you to be heard? How can you go about making sure that you are heard in those situations?
7. What are some other situations or relationships in which it might be important for you to be a good listener? How can you go about making sure that you are using effective listening skills in those situations?
8. If someone asks you for help/understanding/something else, how do you decide whether you want to (or can) meet that need?
9. If you decide you can't meet someone else's need, how do you handle that?
10. What are some other situations in your life in which trusting others is important? How can you apply what you learned about trusting others in this activity to those other situations?
11. In what kind of situation in your life do you decide to be a leader? How do you go about leading? In what kind of situation in your life do you decide to be a follower? How do you go about following? In what kind of situation in your life do you decide to be an observer? How do you go about observing?
12. What are some situations or relationships in which you feel that it is really important to act in a responsible manner? How do you handle these situations or relationships?
13. What are some times when you do not act as responsibly as you think you should? What do you think keeps you from being responsible in those situations? How could you handle those situations differently in the future?
14. How do you feel when you get feedback that you are not acting in a responsible manner? How do you react to this feedback? How is your reaction affected by who it is that is giving the feedback?
15. How do you handle situations in which friends or family members are not acting responsibly? What kinds of feedback do you usually give in these situations? How do you handle situations in which acquaintances or strangers are not acting responsibly? What kinds of feedback do you usually give in these situations?
16. In what kinds of situations in your life do you feel the same kind of stress you felt during this activity? How can you apply what you learned about how you handle stress in this activity to those other situations?
17. What are some other situations in your life in which it is important to exercise self-control and self-discipline? How can you apply what you learned during this activity about your ability to exercise self-control and self-discipline to these situations?
18. What are some other situations in your life in which a person's willingness to act in a responsible manner can affect your ability to trust him or her?

Safety Concerns: Obviously there are all sorts of risks for tripping, etc. This is especially true if your leaders are not attentive, or mindful of safety, and are inclined to think that others bumping into things is funny— in which case we choose another activity.

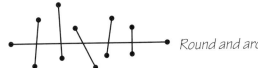 *Round and around, like a Turnstile*

Name of Activity: Turnstiles

Type of Activity: Challenge/Initiative

Grade Level: Third grade and up

Size of Group: 8 to 16

Goal 1: Improve Communication and Relationship Skills

Objectives:

1H.   Recognize and deal with peer pressure
1I.   Use communication skills to resolve conflict
1J.   Recognize the need for help and develop the ability to ask for it
1K.   Recognize and verbalize needs and wishes
1L.   Develop skills for effectively participating in groups

Goal 2: Increase Self-Awareness and Self-Acceptance

Objectives:

2C.   Develop ability to recognize negative self-talk
2D.   Develop skills in replacing negative self-talk with positive self-talk
2F.   Develop positive attitudes toward self

Goal 4: Increase Understanding and Valuing of Diversity

Objectives:

4A.   Recognize and appreciate individual differences
4E.   Recognize how stereotypes can affect interpersonal relationships and attitudes toward others

Goal 5: Demonstrate Consistently Responsible Behavior

Objectives:

5A.   Acknowledge personal responsibilities
5D.   Develop coping skills for dealing with stress
5E.   Understand the need for self-discipline and self-control and how to exercise them

Materials: One jump rope at least 10 to 12 yards long (We like to use old rock-climbing rope, but any easily turned rope will do.)

Preparation: None

How to Play:

1.   This is based on a game of jump rope. As a result, you'll need two turners. Usually we act as one of the turners and have a coleader (if you're lucky enough to have one) or a participant act as the other turner. Sometimes it is also fun to have two participants turn the rope.
2.   Have the turners begin to twirl the jump rope (in the usual way), and tell the group they must get everyone in the group to move through the jump rope (between the two turners) in one of the following ways. Use as few or as many of these methods as you want.
     a.   Have the whole group get over the rope in whatever way they can. Note this is simply letting them all try to get over the rope and through to the other side with no pressure on time.
     b.   Have the group see what is the fewest number of rotations of the jump rope that it takes to get the whole group over.

c. Have the group move through with the stipulation that each person must jump once, rather than simply running through, before exiting the jumping area (where the rope is touching the ground).

d. Have the group send one person running through for every single rotation of the jump rope. (Every time the rope turns, another person runs through).

e. Have the whole group get in the middle and see how many jumps they can complete as a group. Have them try to beat their own record.

f. Have participants run through one at a time. However, every time someone goes through the jump rope he or she must call the person that goes next by name without allowing the jumping area to be empty for one full rotation (pretty tricky).

g. Have the group work together to pass a certain number of balls or balloons through the jump rope as the group moves through the jumping area.

h. Make up some new variations and send them to us!

Variations:

1. Make the stipulation that if anyone in the group does not make it through the jump rope (e.g., trips over the rope and so stops the rotation of the jump rope, breaks the rules by letting two rotations pass if that was the variation being played), the entire group must start the activity again.

2. Asking for volunteers to twirl the rope can be a gracious out for some group members who want to be involved but who don't want to jump. Remember to be sensitive to the challenge by choice philosophy while still encouraging active participation wherever possible.

3. Have group members twirl the rope as well as have to get through the rope with the rest of the group.

4. For large groups, have three ropes that form a large triangle. Place everyone in the group in the middle of the three ropes. Have all three ropes twirling at the same time and explain that everyone must exit the enclosed area through one of the twirling ropes. Complicated—but fun!

Sample Personalization-Processing Questions:

1. What did you feel/think about the group's chances for success when the leader first explained the rules? How did you express your thoughts and feelings? How did your initial attitude affect your approach to solving the problem?

2. If you had trouble jumping the rope, how was that for you? Did you define your difficulties as a failure? If you did, how did you handle this failure? What did you tell yourself about yourself and your abilities related to this failure? What did you tell yourself about the other group members related to this failure? How could you have dealt with this more constructively?

3. If you jumped the rope easily, with no problem, how was that for you? Did you define this as a success? If so, how did you handle this success? What did you tell yourself about yourself and your abilities related to this success? What did you tell yourself about the other group members related to this success? Was there some way you could have dealt with this more constructively?

4. What role did trust play in this activity? What could you have done to enhance trust between the members of the group? What could other group members have done to enhance trust?

5. How could you tell whether you needed more help from the other members of the group? What did you do when you needed more help? How did you ask for more help when you recognized you needed it?

6. Did you accept help/suggestions from others if they offered it? How could you enhance your ability to accept help/suggestions from others?

7. How did your approach to this activity differ from the other members' approaches? How was your approach similar to the approaches of the other group members?

8. Was there any conflict during the process? How did you feel about the conflict? What did you do about your feelings? How did you deal with the conflict? What would have been some other (perhaps more constructive) ways to do this?

9. What were your responsibilities in this activity? How did you decide what your responsibilities were?

10. Did you honor those responsibilities in playing this activity? If yes, what kinds of things did you do that you felt were responsible? How did you make sure your behavior was responsible? If no, what kinds of things did you do that you felt were not responsible? What kept you from being more responsible?
11. Were there times when you were telling yourself negative things about your ability to jump the rope? What kinds of things were you telling yourself?
12. How could you have changed this negative self-talk to more positive self-talk? What kinds of positive things could you tell yourself?
13. What part did self-control and self-discipline play in this activity? How could you have exercised more self-control and self-discipline?
14. What part did peer pressure play in this activity? How did you cope with any peer pressure you felt? Did you pressure any of the other people in the group? What strategies could you have used to improve your ability to cope with peer pressure?
15. Did you notice any stereotypes you were holding about certain people during this activity? How did your holding those stereotypes affect your participation or interaction with others in the group?
16. How stressful was this activity for you? If it was stressful, what made it stressful for you? How could you have improved your ability to deal with this stress?

Sample Application-Processing Questions:

1. In what other situations or relationships in your life does it feel as though you have to jump through hoops? What resources/strategies do you have to help you deal with these situations?
2. What part does cooperation play in these situations or relationships? How do you elicit cooperation and help?
3. What are some other situations in which you might need to ask for help? How can you go about recognizing that you need help and asking for it? What are some other situations in which you might need to ask for what you want and/or need? How can you go about recognizing that you want and/or need something and asking for it?
4. How can you apply some of the methods for appropriately resolving conflicts that you learned/practiced in this activity in other situations?
5. How can you apply what you learned about dealing with negative self-talk?
6. What are some other situations in your life in which taking responsibility and/or being responsible is important? How can you apply what you learned in this activity about taking responsibility and/or being responsible to those other situations?
7. What are some other situations in your life in which trusting others is important? How can you apply what you learned in this activity about trusting others to those other situations?
8. What are some other situations in which you have felt like a success? How have you handled these situations? How can you apply what you learned in this activity to those situations?
9. What are some other situations in which you have felt like a failure? How have you handled these situations? How can you apply what you learned in this activity to those situations?
10. What are some other situations or relationships in which you compare yourself to others? What has the impact of those comparisons been on you and/or your relationships? How can you apply what you learned in this activity about comparing yourself to others to those situations or relationships?
11. What are some other situations in your life in which recognizing and coping with peer pressure is important? How can you apply what you learned in this activity about recognizing and dealing with peer pressure to those other situations?
12. What are some other situations in your life in which self-control and self-discipline is important? How can you apply what you learned in this activity about self-control and self-discipline to those other situations?
13. How can stereotypes affect your interpersonal relationships and attitudes toward others? What are some things you can do to prevent this from happening? How can you become more consistently respectful toward other people?

Safety Concerns: Play on a soft area (i.e., grass) if possible. Participants can trip and fall (not that we've ever done that).

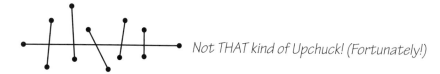

Name of Activity: Upchuck

Type of Activity: Challenge/Initiative

Grade Level: Fifth grade and up

Size of Group: 8 to 40

Goal 1: Improve Communication and Relationship Skills

Objectives:

- 1D. Express ideas clearly and constructively
- 1E. Listen actively to others
- 1G. Develop skills for making and maintaining relationships
- 1H. Recognize and deal with peer pressure
- 1J. Recognize the need for help and develop the ability to ask for it
- 1K. Recognize and verbalize needs and wishes
- 1L. Develop skills for effectively participating in groups

Goal 2: Increase Self-Awareness and Self-Acceptance

Objectives:

- 2C. Develop ability to recognize negative self-talk
- 2D. Develop skills in replacing negative self-talk with positive self-talk
- 2F. Develop positive attitudes toward self
- 2H. Identify personal and social roles

Goal 3: Develop and Apply Problem-Solving and Decision-Making Skills

Objectives:

- 3A. Set personal goals
- 3B. Identify problems
- 3C. Demonstrate understanding of steps for solving problems and making decisions (gather information; explore alternatives and consequences; plan and take action)
- 3D. Evaluate decisions
- 3E. Manage change and transitions in everyday life
- 3J. Develop ability to identify alternative methods for solving problems and achieving goals

Materials: Soft ball or throwable object for each participant

Preparation: None

How to Play:

1. The object of this activity is to have each participant throw his or her ball in the air and make sure that all the balls are caught—with the provision that no participant can catch the same object he or she threw.
2. Have the group members stand in a circle or cluster or however the group wants to configure itself.
3. Before you start the real activity, we like to practice a bit. Ask everyone to toss their balls about 10 feet in the air and then attempt to catch their own balls. We like to practice this skill for two or three tosses.
4. After you are sure that everyone has the hang of this throwing up and catching thing, explain to the group that, on the next toss, everyone has to toss their ball into the air and catch a ball they did not throw.

5. After the toss and attempted catches, count the number of balls that the group was not able to catch. We often like to challenge the group to see if they can have a round where fewer balls are dropped to the floor or even that all the balls are caught (remembering that the thrower cannot catch the same ball he or she threw).[1]

Variations:

1. Start the group by throwing one ball aloft and having someone different catch it. On the next round, throw two balls, and so on until all the balls have been thrown simultaneously and caught. If a ball is missed, the group can start over with one ball being lofted.
2. Instead of a ball-shaped object, use other soft or light objects that can be flung airborne!

Sample Personalization-Processing Questions:

1. What was fun for you in this activity? How did you express your feelings related to having fun? What was challenging to you? How did you handle the things that were challenging for you?
2. How successful was your group with this activity? How did you define success? Did the different members of your group define success differently? How did these differences affect the communication and cooperation in the group?
3. If your group failed, how was that for you? How did you handle this failure? What did you tell yourself about yourself and your abilities related to this failure? What did you tell yourself about other members of your group related to this failure? How could you have dealt with this more constructively?
4. If your group was successful, how was that for you? How did you handle this success? What did you tell yourself about yourself and your abilities related to this success? What did you tell yourself about other members of your group related to this success?
5. If there were a number of small groups doing this activity, did you compare your group to other groups? What effect did this comparison have on you? Did you compare yourself to the other members of your group? What effect did this comparison have on you?
6. How important was communication between you and the other members of your group in this activity?
7. Did you feel heard by the other members of your group as you worked on throwing and catching the objects? Did you feel heard by the other members of your group if you stopped to strategize? If you did feel heard, how was that for you? If you didn't feel heard, how was that for you?
8. If you only felt heard some of the time, what do you think determined whether you were heard? If you had wanted to be heard more consistently by the other members of the group, what could you have done differently to make sure that you were heard?
9. Did you communicate your ideas effectively? Did you communicate your needs and wishes effectively? If so, how did you go about doing this? If not, what prevented you from doing this? How could you go about communicating your ideas, needs, and wishes more effectively?
10. Why was listening important in this activity? How did you do as a listener in this activity? How could you have improved your listening?
11. What process did the members of the group use to determine how to go about throwing and catching the object? How did the members of the group decide whether a strategy was working? If a strategy wasn't working, how did the group deal with that? How did you go about developing an alternative strategy when something wasn't working?
12. If the members of the group kept dropping the objects, how did you apply what you learned from these mistakes to perfect what the group was doing?
13. Why was cooperation important in this activity? What were some of the ways that the members of the group cooperated with one another to accomplish this task? How did cooperation help?
14. How did you decide whether to cooperate or not? How did your attitudes about cooperation influence what happened among the members of the group?
15. How could you tell whether you needed more help from the other members of the group? What did you do when you needed more help? How did you ask for more help when you recognized you needed it?
16. What role did you play in this process (leader? follower? observer?)? Did the group need someone to be the leader to be able to throw and catch the objects? If so, how did you work out who was going to lead and who was going to follow? Did the roles change during the course of the activity? How?

---

[1]*Note.* Adapted from Rohnke, K., & Butler, S. (1995). *Quicksilver.* Dubuque, IA: Kendall Hunt.

17. If group members disagreed on strategies for throwing and catching the objects, did you define that disagreement as conflict? If yes, how did you feel about the conflict? What did you do about your feelings? How did the members of the group resolve the conflict? What would have been some other ways to do this?

18. How did you feel about it when the group was able to throw the objects and they were all caught?

19. How did you react when other people had different ideas? How did you decide which ideas were ideas the group should try?

20. On a 1 to 10 scale, how stressful was this activity for you? What made it stressful? Where did you feel the stress in your body? What could you have done to make the activity less stressful for you?

21. Were there any instances in which peer pressure affected the group members during this process? What impact did peer pressure have on you? What did you do to cope with peer pressure?

22. How did you decide which object to catch? What happened if the object you chose was difficult to catch?

23. How did you feel if you dropped the ball? What did you tell yourself about your abilities when/if you dropped the ball? If you were using negative self-talk, how could you switch it to more positive self-talk?

Sample Application-Processing Questions:

1. In what other situations or relationships in your life does it feel as though you must work with other people to make something happen? What resources/strategies do you have to help you deal with these situations?

2. What part does cooperation play in these situations or relationships? How do you elicit cooperation and help?

3. In other situations in your life, how do you decide what role you are going to play?

4. How do you usually go about solving problems? Which of the methods for problem solving used by the members of the group would be useful in other situations in your life? How can you use them in these situations?

5. What are some other situations in which you might need to ask for help? How can you go about recognizing that you need help and asking for it?

6. What are some other situations or relationships in which it might be important for you to be heard? How can you go about making sure that you are heard in those situations?

7. What are some other situations or relationships in which it might be important for you to be a good listener? How can you go about making sure that you are using effective listening skills in those situations?

8. What are some other situations or relationships in which you need to use your conflict resolution skills? How can you apply some of the methods that you learned/practiced in this activity for appropriately resolving conflicts in these situations?

9. What are some other situations in which you have felt like you had failed? How have you handled these situations? How can you apply what you learned in this activity to those situations?

10. What are some other situations or relationships in which you compare yourself to others? What has the impact of those comparisons been on you and/or your relationships? How can you apply what you learned in this activity about comparing yourself to others to those situations or relationships?

11. In what kind of situation in your life do you decide to be a leader? How do you go about leading? In what kind of situation in your life do you decide to be a follower? How do you go about following? In what kind of situation in your life do you decide to be an observer? How do you go about observing?

12. Do you ever experience your life as a series of objects thrown up in the air that have to be caught? How do you cope in those situations? What did you learn from playing this activity that might help in those situations?

13. What are some situations in your life in which you feel as if you dropped the ball? How have you handled those situations in the past? What have you learned from this activity that would help you handle those situations better in the future?

Safety Concerns: Make sure the ball is soft (e.g., Nerf ball, beach ball, sock ball) or the object is light (e.g., plastic lid, Frisbee).

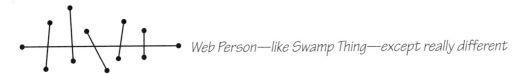

Name of Activity: Web Person

Type of Activity: *Trust; Challenge/Initiative*

Grade Level: *Seventh grade and up*

Size of Group: *8 to 15*

Goal 1: Improve Communication and Relationship Skills

Objectives:

1C.   Recognize and accept the feelings of others
1D.   Express ideas clearly and constructively
1F.   Demonstrate willingness to trust others
1G.   Develop skills for making and maintaining relationships
1L.   Develop skills for effectively participating in groups

Goal 2: Increase Self-Awareness and Self-Acceptance

Objectives:

2B.   Identify and acknowledge personal positive traits, talents, and accomplishments
2C.   Develop ability to recognize negative self-talk
2D.   Develop skills in replacing negative self-talk with positive self-talk
2F.   Develop positive attitudes toward self
2G.   Recognize personal boundaries, rights, and privacy needs

Goal 5: Demonstrate Consistently Responsible Behavior

Objectives:

5A.   Acknowledge personal responsibilities
5C.   Act in an appropriate and responsible manner
5D.   Develop coping skills for dealing with stress
5E.   Understand the need for self-discipline and self-control and how to exercise them

Goal 6: Enhance Positive Attitudes and Skills Related to Learning

Objectives:

6A.   Develop feeling of competence and confidence as a learner
6B.   Take pride in accomplishments
6C.   Accept mistakes as part of the learning process
6D.   Apply time management and task management strategies
6E.   Recognize that effort and persistence enhance learning
6F.   Demonstrate dependability and initiative
6G.   Develop the ability to share knowledge
6H.   Develop critical-thinking skills

Materials: A long piece of 1–inch tubular webbing rolled into a ball (like a ball of yarn). The webbing should be long enough to account for at least 5 to 6 feet of webbing for each person within the group. Tubular webbing can be purchased at most outdoor recreation equipment stores and is relatively inexpensive.

Preparation: None

How to Play:

1. Explain to the group that the objective of this activity is for the group to lift and move a student using the long piece of 1–inch webbing.
2. Have the group members stand in a circle (shoulder to shoulder, facing inward).
3. Ask one person to volunteer to be carried by the group and have that person step outside the circle.
4. Have one of the group members standing in the circle hold the end of the webbing and toss the rest of the webbing to someone across the circle. The second person should grasp the webbing with a two-handed grip, and while maintaining his or her grip toss the rest of the webbing to another person across the circle. This process continues until everyone is gripping a piece of the webbing, which forms a web in the middle of the group.
5. Once everyone is holding the webbing, continue to toss the now diminishing ball of webbing around the circle, continuing to develop the web.
6. After all of the webbing has been used, have the group kneel down and place the web on the ground.
7. Have the group member who has been outside of the circle adjust the web to his or her liking/satisfaction. In addition, encourage the participant to give the group some feedback about their process and/or ask for anything the participant might need (e.g., verbal encouragement like "we've got you!") to feel comfortable.
8. Have the participant lie down face up on the web.
9. After the group member is lying on the web, have the group holding the web stand and lift the person off the ground.
10. Have the group transport the participant on the web some designated distance before lowering him or her to the ground again—what a ride!
11. Depending on the time frame more than one person can take the ride. (To do this we usually have the participant who has just ridden simply change places with the next rider. It can also be fun to process a little in between riders).

Variations:

1. Problem-solving variation: Give the group the materials and tell them they must move one member of the group a specified distance without physically touching the group member.
2. Possible follow-up activity: The web can be used to symbolize how everyone in the group is connected and that in order to be successful the whole group must remain focused and work together. To highlight this point after moving a group member and laying him or her back on the ground, have the person stay on the web and ask one person of the group to let go of the webbing and see if the rest of the group can still pick up the person using the web.
3. Additional follow-up activity: Have each group member identify one unique attribute they bring to the group in order to help the group succeed.

Sample Personalization-Processing Questions:

1. What was your reaction when you first heard the directions to this activity? How did you express your thoughts and feelings? Did your reaction change as the group discussed strategies? How?
2. What did you do to contribute to the success of the group? How did you feel about your contribution?
3. If you were one of the people who got carried, how did that feel? What was fun about it? What made that fun for you? What was scary/challenging about it? What made that scary/challenging for you?
4. What role did trust play in this activity?
5. If you were one of the people being carried, how did you decide whether to trust the people who were arranging and holding the web? What would have increased your level of trust/sense of safety?
6. If you were one of the people being carried, how did you decide whether to rearrange the web before you lay down on the web?
7. If you were one of the people being carried, what kind of feedback did you give to the rest of the group before you were carried on the web?
8. If you were one of the people being carried, what did you ask for from the rest of the group? How did you decide what to ask for? How comfortable were you with asking for what you wanted and needed?

9. When you were one of the people arranging and holding the web, what did you do to enhance the feelings of trust and safety of the person you were going to carry?
10. Why was being responsible important in this activity?
11. What process did the members of the group use to determine how to go about deciding how to arrange and hold the web? How did the group members decide whether a strategy was working? If a strategy wasn't working, how did the group members deal with that? How did you go about developing an alternative strategy when something wasn't working?
12. As the group members discussed how to arrange the web and their strategy for carrying folks, did you feel heard by the other members of the group? How did it feel when you were heard by other members of the group?
13. If you didn't feel heard, what was that like for you? If you had wanted to be heard by the other members of the group, what could you have done differently to make sure that you were heard?
14. Did you communicate your ideas and feelings effectively? If so, how did you go about doing this? If not, what prevented you from doing this?
15. What did you do to make sure that everyone who wanted to be heard was heard?
16. If the webbing started to slip, how did you use what you learned from this mistake to do a better job arranging and holding the web?
17. What were some of the ways that group members cooperated with one another to accomplish this task? Why was cooperation necessary?
18. How did you decide whether to cooperate or not? How did your attitudes about cooperation influence what happened in the group? What about the attitudes of other group members?
19. As you carried the webbing with the person riding on it, how could you tell whether you needed help from other group members? What did you do when you needed help? How did you ask for help when you recognized you needed it?
20. How did you feel about being physically close and/or touching one another as you carried the person in the webbing? How much personal space do you need? How is this different from the other people in the group and their personal space requirements?
21. What was your level of stress during this activity? What was stressful about this activity? What strategies did you use to cope with the stress involved in this activity?
22. In what ways did peer pressure affect the process? How did the members of your group handle the peer pressure?
23. What were your responsibilities to the group in this activity? What were your responsibilities to the person who was being carried? How did you decide what your responsibilities were?
24. Did you honor those responsibilities during this activity? If yes, what kinds of things did you do that you felt were responsible? How did you make sure your behavior was responsible? If not, what kinds of things did you do that you felt were not responsible? What kept you from being more responsible?
25. Were there times when you were telling yourself negative things about your ability to make a contribution to the group's success? What kinds of things were you telling yourself?
26. How could you have changed this negative self-talk to more positive self-talk? What kinds of positive things could you tell yourself?
27. What role did dependability and initiative play in this activity? Why was it important for all of the members of the group to be dependable? How dependable were you? How did you decide whether to be dependable or not?

Sample Application-Processing Questions:

1. What are other situations or relationships in your life in which it feels as though you must carry others? What resources/strategies do you have to help you deal with these situations?
2. What are other situations or relationships in your life in which it feels as though you must be carried by others? What resources/strategies do you have to help you deal with these situations?
3. What are some other situations in your life in which you must have cooperation and help (work as a team) to be successful? How do you deal with these situations? How do you elicit cooperation and help?

4. How do you go about solving problems that are similar to the situation in this activity? Which of the methods for problem solving used by the members of your group would be useful in other situations in your life? How can you use them in those situations?
5. Which of the methods for managing stress that you or the members of your group used would be helpful in other situations in your life? How can you use them?
6. What are some other situations in which you might need to ask for help? How can you go about recognizing that you need help and asking for it?
7. What are some other situations or relationships in which it might be important for you to be heard? How can you go about making sure that you are heard in those situations?
8. How can you apply some of the methods for communicating about feelings and ideas, encouraging cooperation, solving problems, and/or appropriately resolving conflicts that you learned/practiced in this activity in other situations?
9. How can you apply what you learned about dealing with negative self-talk? Dealing with peer pressure?
10. What could you learn from this game that you could apply in situations in which it would be important to recognize and maintain your personal boundaries, rights, and privacy needs?
11. What are the rules (spoken or unspoken) about personal space and/or touching in your family? In your culture?
12. What did you learn about your critical-thinking skills that you can apply to other situations in your life?
13. What are some other situations in your life in which taking responsibility is important? How can you apply what you learned about taking responsibility in this activity to those other situations?
14. What are some other situations in your life in which trusting others is important? How can you apply what you learned about trusting others in this activity to those other situations?

Safety Concerns:

1. Instruct group on proper lifting techniques. They should be sure to lift bending their legs rather than their backs (e.g., kneeling down vs. bending over), maintain a nice wide stance with their feet, and hold on to the webbing with both hands.
2. Monitor to make sure the group is focused.
3. Maintain the carried person's head higher than other portions of his or her body.
4. Complete activity over grass or other soft surface.

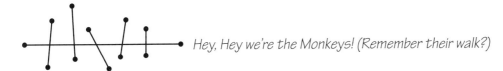

Hey, Hey we're the Monkeys! (Remember their walk?)

Name of Activity: Welded Ankles

Type of Activity: Challenge/Initiative

Grade Level: Fifth grade and up

Size of Group: 10 to 20

Goal 1: Improve Communication and Relationship Skills

Objectives:

1B.   Express feelings clearly and constructively
1C.   Recognize and accept the feelings of others
1D.   Express ideas clearly and constructively
1E.   Listen actively to others
1G.   Develop skills for making and maintaining relationships
1H.   Recognize and deal with peer pressure
1I.   Use communication skills to resolve conflict
1J.   Recognize the need for help and develop the ability to ask for it
1K.   Recognize and verbalize needs and wishes
1L.   Develop skills for effectively participating in groups

Goal 2: Increase Self-Awareness and Self-Acceptance

Objectives:

2B.   Identify and acknowledge personal positive traits, talents, and accomplishments
2C.   Develop ability to recognize negative self-talk
2D.   Develop skills in replacing negative self-talk with positive self-talk
2F.   Develop positive attitudes toward self
2G.   Recognize personal boundaries, rights, and privacy needs
2H.   Identify personal and social roles

Goal 3: Develop and Apply Problem-Solving and Decision-Making Skills

Objectives:

3A.   Set personal goals
3B.   Identify problems
3C.   Demonstrate understanding of steps for solving problems and making decisions (gather information; explore alternatives and consequences; plan and take action)
3D.   Evaluate decisions
3F.   Apply decision-making skills to resolve conflicts
3G.   Apply decision-making skills in life situations
3H.   Demonstrate effective coping skills for dealing with problems
3I.   Recognize when peer pressure is influencing decision making
3J.   Develop ability to identify alternative methods for solving problems and achieving goals

Goal 5: Demonstrate Consistently Responsible Behavior

Objectives:

5A.   Acknowledge personal responsibilities
5B.   Recognize whether behavior is appropriate and responsible

5C. Act in an appropriate and responsible manner
5D. Develop coping skills for dealing with stress
5E. Understand the need for self-discipline and self-control and how to exercise them
5G. Demonstrate respect for alternate perspectives

Goal 6: Enhance Positive Attitudes and Skills Related to Learning

Objectives:

6B. Take pride in accomplishments
6C. Accept mistakes as part of the learning process
6D. Apply time management and task management strategies
6E. Recognize that effort and persistence enhance learning
6F. Demonstrate dependability and initiative
6G. Develop the ability to share knowledge
6H. Develop critical-thinking skills

Materials: None

Preparation: Mark out an open area for the group to try to cross. (We usually use 20 to 40 feet.)

How to Play:

1. This is a simple activity in which the group must walk together, with completely coordinated steps, across an open area. Sounds easy—not so much.
2. Ask the participants to stand in a straight line facing you with the sides of their feet or shoes touching the sides of the feet or shoes of the participants on both sides of them. Note that the two people on the ends of the line will only have one foot connected to the feet of other participants.
3. Explain to the group that the object of this activity is for the group to move across the designated open area as a group and that they must do so staying connected by maintaining contact with the sides of their shoes or feet (i.e., as if their ankles were welded together). Also explain that, if contact is lost, the group must begin again.

Variations:

Have the group stand in a circle with feet touching. Have the group imagine they are a clock and need to move the person at 12:00 to the 6:00 position without anyone losing contact with their feet.

Sample Personalization-Processing Questions:

1. What was the most fun aspect of this activity for you? How did you express your feelings to the rest of the group?
2. What was the most challenging/frustrating aspect of this activity for you? How did you express your feelings to the rest of the group? What did you do to deal with your frustrations? How could you have dealt with your frustrations in a more appropriate way?
3. What would have made the activity less challenging/frustrating for you?
4. If your group did successfully cross the space, how did you feel about that success? What did you do to contribute to the successful crossing? How did you feel about your contribution?
5. If your group had to start over, how did you feel about that? What did you tell yourself about your abilities if you were one of the people whose ankles came unwelded, causing the group to have to start over? If what you told yourself was negative, what else could you have told yourself that was more positive?
6. If you were one of the people whose ankles came unwelded, how did you handle that mistake? How could you have handled it better? What did you learn from that mistake? How did you apply what you learned from that mistake to future attempts to cross the space?
7. Did your group develop a strategy for crossing the space? If not, how did that work for you? What do you wish the group members had done?
8. If your group did develop a strategy, what process did the members of the group use to determine how to go about keeping their ankles welded as they crossed the space? How did the group members decide whether a strategy was working? If a strategy wasn't working, how did

the group members deal with that? How did you go about developing an alternative strategy when something wasn't working?

9. Did you communicate your ideas and feelings effectively? If so, how did you go about doing this? If not, what prevented you from doing this?

10. What were some of the ways that group members cooperated with one another to accomplish this task? What made cooperation necessary for accomplishing this task?

11. How did you decide whether to cooperate or not? How did your attitudes about cooperation influence what happened in the group? What about the attitudes of other group members?

12. How could you have been better at communicating with other group members? How could you have been more cooperative?

13. How could you tell whether you needed help from other group members? What did you do when you needed help? How did you ask for help when you recognized you needed it? If you didn't ask for help, what prevented you from doing this?

14. Was it necessary for the group to have a leader to be successful in this activity? If no leader emerged, how did the members of the group handle this? If a leader did emerge, how did that happen?

15. How did you feel about being physically close and/or touching one another as you crossed the space? How much personal space do you need? How is this different from the other people in the group and their personal space requirements?

16. What did you communicate to the rest of the group when mistakes happened?

17. If you were not one of the people who messed up, how did you feel about having to start over again even though you had not messed up? How did you express your feelings to the group?

18. What was your level of stress during this activity? How did it change as the number of times you had to start over mounted? If you had a time limit, how did this affect your stress level? What strategies did you use to cope with the stress involved in this activity?

19. When members of the group disagreed on strategies for keeping their ankles welded and crossing the space, how did you feel about the disagreement? What did you do about your feelings? Did you feel that the disagreement was a conflict? How do you decide whether a situation is a conflict? If there was a conflict, how did the group members resolve it? What would have been some other ways to do this?

20. In what ways did peer pressure affect the process? How was peer pressure expressed/exerted? How did the members of your group handle the peer pressure?

21. What personal positive traits and talents did you bring to this process, and how did you use them to help in keeping ankles welded as you crossed the space?

22. If you were feeling discouraged in this process, how did you deal with that? What did you tell yourself to motivate yourself to continue? If other group members were feeling discouraged, how did you interact with them about their discouragement?

23. What were your responsibilities to the group in this activity? How did you decide what your responsibilities were?

24. What part did effort and persistence have in influencing your group's experience in this activity? Dependability and initiative? Self-discipline and self-control? Respect for alternate perspectives? Critical-thinking skills?

Sample Application-Processing Questions:

1. How do you define success in other situations in your life? How can you apply what you learned in this activity about yourself and the way you think and feel about success to other situations in your life?

2. What are other situations or relationships in your life in which it feels as though the outcome is not in your control? What resources do you have to help you deal with these situations?

3. What are some other situations in your life in which you must have cooperation and help (work as a team) to be successful? How do you deal with these situations? How do you elicit cooperation and help?

4. How do you handle situations in which the chances of success would be enhanced if there was a group leader? How do you respond if there is lack of leadership in these situations? Do you ever step up to be the leader in these situations? How do you decide whether you will do this?

5. Which methods for problem-solving used by the members of your group would be useful in other situations in your life? How can you use them in these situations?

6. Which of the methods for managing stress used by you or the members of your group would be helpful in other situations in your life? How can you use them?

7. What are some other situations in which you might need to ask for help? How can you go about recognizing that you need help and asking for it?

8. How can you apply some of the methods for communicating about feelings and ideas, encouraging cooperation, solving problems, and/or appropriately resolving conflicts that you learned/practiced in this activity in other situations?

9. How can you apply what you learned about dealing with mistakes in other situations? Dealing with negative self-talk? Encouraging persistence and flexibility? Dealing with peer pressure? Exercising self-control and self-discipline? Being dependable and showing initiative? Using self-discipline and self-control? Having respect for alternate perspectives?

10. What could you learn from this activity that you could apply in situations in which it would be important to recognize and maintain your personal boundaries, rights, and privacy needs?

11. What are the rules (spoken or unspoken) about personal space and/or touching in your family? In your culture?

12. What are some other situations in which you have noticed differences in people's comfort levels about personal space and/or physical touch? What were the differences that you noticed? If someone else has different rules than you do about personal space, how can you handle this in an appropriate and respectful way?

13. What did you learn about your critical-thinking skills that you can apply to other situations in your life?

14. What are some other situations in your life in which you could notice and celebrate your own uniqueness? Your talents, abilities, contributions? Your successes?

Safety Concerns: Play on grass or another soft surface as it can be awkward to move and try to keep ankles welded.

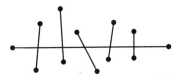

I'm their leader! Which way did they go?

Name of Activity: Who Do You Follow?

Type of Activity: Deinhibitizer

Grade Level: Fifth grade and up

Size of Group: 8 to 25

Goal 2: Increase Self-Awareness and Self-Acceptance

Objectives:

2C.   Develop ability to recognize negative self-talk
2D.   Develop skills in replacing negative self-talk with positive self-talk
2F.   Develop positive attitudes toward self
2H.   Identify personal and social roles

Goal 3: Develop and Apply Problem-Solving and Decision-Making Skills

Objectives:

3D.   Evaluate decisions
3H.   Demonstrate effective coping skills for dealing with problems
3J.   Develop ability to identify alternative methods for solving problems and achieving goals

Goal 6: Enhance Positive Attitudes and Skills Related to Learning

Objectives:

6A.   Develop feeling of competence and confidence as a learner
6B.   Take pride in accomplishments
6C.   Accept mistakes as part of the learning process
6H.   Develop critical-thinking skills

Materials: None

Preparation: None

How to Play:

1.   In this activity, all the participants are following a leader. The participants are doing everything that the leader does. The fun is that one participant doesn't know who the leader is and is trying to figure it out—tricky business.
2.   Have the group form a circle and choose one person who will leave the area (so he or she can't see who the leader is going to be). Note that this can be a strategic choice because of the feeling of being left out and not knowing who the leader is.
3.   Choose a leader from the remaining participants. Everyone will follow this leader throughout the activity. Note that this can also be a strategic choice because of the feeling of everyone else in the group doing exactly what you choose to do. Pretty heady stuff.
4.   Explain to the leader that his or her job is to change motions and postures fairly quickly (making it a little more difficult to identify who the actual leader is). We often encourage large gestures and outlandish movements. More fun and more distracting.
5.   Explain to the rest of the group that their job is to follow the newly chosen leader doing everything that he or she does. Encourage the group members to change their posture as quickly as possible after the leader changes his or hers.
6.   After the leader has been chosen and the group instructions given, the participant who left the area can return.

7. The one participant who was out of the room while the leader was chosen gets three guesses to identify the leader of the group.
8. If the leader is correctly identified or if the guesser runs out of guesses, that round of the game ends and new participants are chosen for each role.

Variations:

1. You can add a competitive or cooperative edge to the game by sending more than one person out of the room to be the guessers, who then can either work together or compete against each other.
2. A silly twist we have used is to actually make the guesser the leader such that the group is doing what that person does. The guesser is leading and, at least initially, doesn't know it.

Sample Personalization-Processing Questions:

1. If you were one of the people who left the room and had to guess who the leader was, how was that process for you? How did you feel when you left the room? How did you feel when you came back and everybody else knew who the leader was and you didn't?
2. If you were a guesser, how did you decide who you thought was the leader? If you guessed wrong, how was that for you? Did you learn from your mistake in the initial guesses and change your strategy for figuring out who the leader was?
3. If you guessed correctly, how did you feel about that? What did you tell yourself about yourself/your abilities if this happened?
4. If you guessed wrong all three times, how did you feel about that? What did you tell yourself about yourself/your abilities if this happened? If you wanted to use more positive self-talk, what could you have told yourself instead?
5. If you were one of the people chosen as the leader, how did it feel to have everyone else doing just what you were doing?
6. If you were one of the people chosen as the leader, how did you feel if the guesser guessed your identity quickly? How did you feel if the guesser never guessed your identity?
7. How did you use critical-thinking skills in this process?
8. What did you learn about yourself during this activity?

Sample Application-Processing Questions:

1. What are some situations in which you must use your critical-thinking skills to figure something out? How can you use what you learned in this activity about yourself and your critical-thinking skills in those situations?
2. What are some situations in which you are the center of attention? How do you feel about being the center of attention? If you are uncomfortable being the center of attention, how could you become more comfortable with that?
3. What are some situations in which you feel left out of the group? How do you feel about those situations?
4. How do you handle it when you feel left out? What is hard for you in those situations? What do you tell yourself about yourself when you feel left out? How do you wish you handled those situations? What could you do differently in those situations that would make the experience more positive/less painful for you?
5. What are some other situations in which you get to be fully expressive with your body? How do you experience those situations? How could you become more comfortable with being fully expressive with your body?
6. In real life, how do you decide who to follow? How do you decide whether to continue to follow that person? What would be some things a person could do that would convince you that it would be wiser to stop following him or her?
7. What are some situations or relationships in which you tend to engage in negative self-talk? What kinds of things do you tell yourself when you are engaging in negative self-talk?
8. How can you get better at recognizing negative self-talk? How can you go about substituting more positive self-talk for that negative self-talk?

Safety Concerns: None

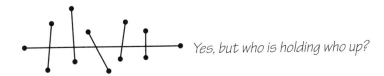 *Yes, but who is holding who up?*

Name of Activity: Yurt Pull

Type of Activity: *Trust*

Grade Level: *Fifth grade and up*

Size of Group: *8 to 40; you just need an even number. Of course, you can also play.*

Goal 1: Improve Communication and Relationship Skills

Objectives:

1B. Express feelings clearly and constructively
1C. Recognize and accept the feelings of others
1E. Listen actively to others
1F. Demonstrate willingness to trust others
1G. Develop skills for making and maintaining relationships
1K. Recognize and verbalize needs and wishes
1L. Develop skills for effectively participating in groups

Goal 5: Demonstrate Consistently Responsible Behavior

Objectives:

5A. Acknowledge personal responsibilities
5B. Recognize whether behavior is appropriate and responsible
5C. Act in an appropriate and responsible manner
5D. Develop coping skills for dealing with stress
5E. Understand the need for self-discipline and self-control and how to exercise them

Materials: None

Preparation: None

How to Play:

1. This activity is a great cooperative leaning activity.
2. To begin, have the participants (again, remember you need an even number) form a large circle.
3. After participants have formed a circle, have the participants count off by twos around the circle.
4. Have all of the ones face toward the middle of the circle, and the twos face the outside of the circle.
5. Have everyone join hands in a circle. (Note that every other person is facing the opposite direction).
6. Explain to the group that, on the count of three, each participant is to lean back while continuing to hold hands. Every other person in the circle will be leaning in a different direction and, as a result, holding the other participants up. We often think that it looks like a human zigzag chain with people supporting each other.
7. Count to three and watch the magic.
8. When everyone is balanced, explain that when you count to three again participants should stand up straight again (rather than leaning).
9. Count to three and participants should come back to a normal standing position.

Variations:

1. If the group has enjoyed the activity, have them tighten their circle. The closer participants are to each other in the circle, the greater the angle of their lean.
2. After a group has successfully leaned back, have them try leaning forward.

Sample Personalization-Processing Questions:

1. What did you feel/think about your chances for success when the leader first explained the rules? How did you express your thoughts and feelings?
2. What did you do to contribute to the successful lean? How did you feel about your contribution?
3. How important was communication between you and the other members of the group in this activity?
4. Did you communicate your ideas and feelings effectively? Did you communicate your needs and wishes effectively? If so, how did you go about doing this? If not, what prevented you from doing this?
5. How did you do as a listener in this activity? How could you have improved your listening?
6. What role did trust play in this activity? What could you have done to enhance trust?
7. What were some of the ways that you and the other members of the group cooperated with one another to accomplish this task? Why was cooperation necessary?
8. What were your responsibilities to the rest of the group in this activity? How did you decide what your responsibilities were?
9. Did you honor those responsibilities in this activity? If yes, what kinds of things did you do that you felt were responsible? How did you make sure your behavior was responsible? If no, what kinds of things did you do that you felt were not responsible? What kept you from being more responsible?
10. How could you tell whether other people in the group perceived your behaviors as responsible? What kinds of feedback did you get from others (other people in the group, the leader) about whether you were being responsible during this activity? How did you react when you got this kind of feedback?
11. Did you feel that the other people in the group were being responsible during this activity? What kind of feedback did you give others in the group if they were not being responsible during this activity?
12. How did the members in the group and their ability to act in a responsible way affect your ability to trust them?
13. What did you find stressful in this activity? What strategies did you use to cope with this stress? What would have helped to make this activity less stressful for you?
14. Why was it important to exercise self-discipline and self-control during this activity? What was your level of self-discipline and self-control? How could you have exercised more self-discipline and self-control?

Sample Application-Processing Questions:

1. In what other situations or relationships in your life does it feels as though you must work with other people to make something happen? What resources/strategies do you have to help you deal with these situations?
2. What part does cooperation play in these situations or relationships? How do you elicit cooperation from others?
3. What are some other situations in your life in which taking responsibility is important? How can you apply what you learned about taking responsibility in this activity to those other situations?
4. What are some other situations in your life in which trusting others is important? How can you apply what you learned about trusting others in this activity to those other situations?
5. What are some times when you do not act as responsibly as you think you should? What do you think keeps you from being responsible in those situations? How could you handle those situations differently in the future?
6. How do you feel when you get feedback that you are not acting responsibly? How do you react to this feedback? How is your reaction affected by who it is that is giving the feedback? How could you improve your reaction to this kind of feedback?
7. How do you handle situations in which friends or family members are not acting responsibly? What kinds of feedback do you usually give in these situations? How do you handle situations in which acquaintances or strangers are not acting responsibly? What kinds of feedback do you usually give in these situations? How could you learn to be more helpful when you give feedback to others?

8. In what kinds of situations in your life do you feel the same kind of stress you felt during this activity? How can you apply what you learned in this activity about how you handle stress to those other situations?

9. What are some other situations in your life in which it is important to exercise self-control and self-discipline? How can you apply what you learned during this activity about self-control and self-discipline to these situations?

10. What are some other situations in your life in which a person's willingness to act in a responsible manner can affect your ability to trust him or her? How does a person's willingness to act in a responsible manner affect your ability to trust him or her?

Safety Concerns: Be sure to use an even number. Play on grass or another soft surface. Make sure participants have turned correctly before counting to three. Allow the group members to talk about any fears and trust issues before and after the activity.

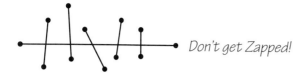

Don't get Zapped!

Name of Activity: Zap

Type of Activity: *Icebreaker*

Grade Level: *Third grade and up*

Size of Group: *2 to 100 (just need an even number—or YOU get to play)*

Goal 1: Improve Communication and Relationship Skills

Objectives:

    1B.   Express feelings clearly and constructively
    1C.   Recognize and accept the feelings of others

Goal 2: Increase Self-Awareness and Self-Acceptance

Objective:

    2G.   Recognize personal boundaries, rights, and privacy needs

Goal 5: Demonstrate Consistently Responsible Behavior

Objectives:

    5B.   Recognize whether behavior is appropriate and responsible
    5C.   Act in an appropriate and responsible manner
    5D.   Develop coping skills for dealing with stress
    5E.   Understand the need for self-discipline and self-control and how to exercise them

Materials: None

Preparation: None

How to Play:

1.   This is a quick, energizing, and somewhat competitive game.
2.   To begin, have everyone find a partner and point at that person (almost like pointing a gun at the person, index finger extended, other fingers in a fist, and thumb raised).
3.   Have each set of partners then interlock their curled fingers, leaving their index finger extended. Note that this looks like a cool handshake with your index finger still extended and pointing at the other person.
4.   The challenge is for participants to try to touch/tag their partner with their extended index finger below their partners' knee while simultaneously preventing their partner from tagging their own leg below the knee (all while keeping their hands connected!).
5.   Set a short time limit of 30 to 90 seconds.
6.   For fun, have those participants congratulate each other and find a new partner to play again!

Variations:

You may want to have participants try this with their eyes closed.

Sample Personalization-Processing Questions:

1.   What was fun about this activity for you? What was challenging/frustrating? How did you express your feelings to your partner(s)? To the group?
2.   Did you react in a competitive way to this activity? How did you express that competitiveness? How could you have expressed your competitiveness in a more constructive way?
3.   Do you find that feeling competitive enhanced your performance or got in your way?

4. What did you find stressful in this activity? What strategies did you use to cope with this stress? What would have made it less stressful for you?
5. How did you feel when/if you got zapped? How did you express your feelings to your partner(s)?
6. How did you feel when/if you were the one who did the zapping? How did you express your feelings to your partner(s)?
7. If you got zapped more than you zapped, how was that for you? How did you handle this failure? What did you tell yourself about yourself and your abilities related to this failure? What did you tell yourself about your partner related to this failure? How could you have dealt with this more constructively?
8. How was it for you to have someone inside your personal space trying to do something to you that you did not want them to do?
9. What did you learn about your personal boundaries, rights, and privacy needs from this experience?
10. How did you react when your partner(s) expressed their feelings during this activity? How did it affect your reaction if their feelings were negative? How did the way they expressed their feelings affect your reaction?
11. What were your responsibilities to your partner in this activity? How did you decide what your responsibilities were?
12. Did you honor those responsibilities to your partner? If yes, what kinds of things did you do that you felt were responsible? How did you make sure your behavior was responsible? If no, what kinds of things did you do that you felt were not responsible? What kept you from being more responsible during this activity?
13. How could you tell whether your partner perceived your behaviors as responsible? What kinds of feedback did you get from your partner about whether you were being responsible during this activity? How did you react when you got this kind of feedback?
14. What about this activity made it important to exercise self-discipline and self-control?

Sample Application-Processing Questions:

1. What are some other situations or relationships in which you feel competitive? How does feeling competitive affect your performance in those situations? Do you find that feeling competitive generally enhances your performance or gets in your way?
2. In what situations is being competitive a positive thing? How can being competitive be a negative experience? What are appropriate ways to express feelings of competitiveness?
3. What could you learn from this activity that you could apply in situations in which it would be important to recognize and maintain your personal boundaries, rights, and privacy needs?
4. What are the rules (spoken or unspoken) about physical touch and/or physical closeness in your family? In your culture?
5. What are some other situations in which you have noticed differences in people's comfort levels about physical touch and/or physical closeness? What were the differences that you noticed? If someone else has rules different from yours about physical touch and/or physical closeness, how can you handle this in an appropriate, respectful way?
6. If someone is invading your personal space or doing something to you that you do not want them to do, how can you handle the situation? How can you make sure that others do not invade your personal space or do things to you that you do not want them to do?
7. What are some situations or relationships when you feel that it is really important to act in a responsible manner? How do you handle these situations or relationships?
8. What are some times when you do not act as responsibly as you think you should? What do you think keeps you from being more responsible in those situations? How could you handle those situations differently in the future?
9. How do you feel when you get feedback that you are not acting in a responsible manner? How do you react to this feedback? How is your reaction affected by who it is that is giving the feedback? By the way the feedback is delivered?
10. What are some other situations in your life in which it is important to exercise self-control and self-discipline? How can you apply what you learned during this activity about your ability to exercise self-control and self-discipline to these situations?

11. What could you learn from this activity that you could apply in situations in which you or others are being/feeling competitive?
12. What did you learn about yourself in this activity?

Safety Concerns: None, except for the potential overenthusiasm of the taggers who could become a little too aggressive.

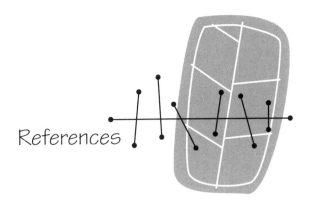

References

American School Counselor Association. (1984). *The school counselor and developmental guidance* (position statement revised from 1978). Alexandria, VA: Author.

American School Counselor Association. (2005). *The ASCA National Model: A framework for school counseling programs* (2nd ed.). Alexandria, VA: Author.

Arlow, J. (2005). Psychoanalysis. In R. Corsini & D. Wedding (Eds.), *Current psychotherapies* (7th ed., pp. 15–51). Belmont, CA: Thompson/Wadsworth.

Baack, S. (1989). *Adventure recreation*. Nashville, TN: Convention Press.

Bandura, A. (1986). *Social foundations of thought and action: A social cognitive theory.* Englewood Cliffs, NJ: Prentice Hall.

Banyai, I. (1995). *Zoom.* New York: Viking/Penguin.

Banyai, I. (1998). *Re-zoom.* New York: Viking/Penguin.

Beaudion, M., & Walden, S. (1998). *Working with groups to enhance relationships.* Duluth, MN: Whole Person Associates.

Beck, A. T. (1976). *Cognitive therapy and the emotional disorders.* New York: International Universities Press.

Bennis, W. (2003). *On becoming a leader.* New York: Basic Books.

Cain, J., & Jolliff, B. (1998). *Teamwork and teamplay.* Dubuque, IA: Kendall Hunt.

Cain, J., & Smith, T. (2002). *The book of raccoon circles.* Dubuque, IA: Kendall Hunt.

Cobb, N. J. (2001). *Adolescence: Continuity, change, and diversity* (4th ed.). Mountain View, CA: Mayfield.

Corey, G. (2007). *Theory and practice of group counseling* (7th ed.). Pacific Grove, CA: Brooks/Cole.

Cornell, J. (1989). *Sharing the joy of nature.* Nevada City, CA: Dawn.

Fluegelman, A. (1976). *The new games book.* San Francisco, CA: New Games Foundation.

Frank, L. (2001). *The caring classroom: Using adventure to create community in the classroom and beyond.* Madison, WI: Goal Consulting.

Gelso, C. J., & Carter, J. A. (1985). The relationship in counseling and psychotherapy: Components, consequences, and theoretical antecedents. *Counseling Psychologist, 13,* 155–243.

Gladding, S. (2002). *Group work: A counseling specialty* (4th ed.). Upper Saddle River, NJ: Merrill.

Hans, T. (2000). A meta-analysis of the effects of adventure programming on locus of control. *Journal of Contemporary Psychotherapy, 30,* 33–60.

Hattie, J., Marsh, H. W., Neill, J. T., & Richards, G. E. (1997). Adventure education and Outward Bound: Out-of-class experiences that make a lasting difference. *Review of Educational Research, 67,* 43–87.

Henton, M. (1996). *Adventure in the classroom.* Dubuque, IA: Kendall Hunt.

Jongsma, A., Peterson, L. M., & McInnis, W. (2002). *The child psychotherapy treatment planner* (3rd ed.). Hoboken, NJ: Wiley.

Jongsma, A., Peterson, L. M., & McInnis, W. (2006). *The adolescent psychotherapy treatment planner* (4th ed.). Hoboken, NJ: Wiley.

Kaplan, P. (2000). *A child's odyssey* (3rd ed.). Belmont, CA: Wadsworth.

Kottman, T. (2001). *Play therapy: Basics and beyond.* Alexandria, VA: American Counseling Association.

Kottman, T. (2002). *Partners in play: An Adlerian approach to play therapy.* Alexandria, VA: American Counseling Association.

Kottman, T., & Ashby, J. S. (2002). Custom designing metaphoric stories for children in play therapy. In C. E. Schaefer & D. M. Cangelosi (Eds.), *Innovative psychotherapy techniques in child and adolescent therapy* (pp. 133–142). New York: Wiley.

Kottman, T., Ashby, J. S., & DeGraaf, D. (2001). *Adventures in guidance: How to integrate fun into your guidance program.* Alexandria, VA: American Counseling Association.

Michaelis, B., & O'Connell, J. (2000). *The game and play leader's handbook.* State College, PA: Venture.

Morris, D., & Stiehl, J. (1989). *Changing kids' games.* Champaign, IL: Human Kinetics.

Muro, J., & Kottman, T. (1995). *Guidance and counseling in the elementary and middle schools: A practical approach.* Dubuque, IA: Brown & Benchmark.

Priest, S., & Rohnke, K. (1999). *101 of the best corporate team-building activities we know.* Dubuque, IA: Kendall Hunt.

Rogers, C. R. (1959). A theory of therapy, personality, and interpersonal relationships, as developed in the client-centered framework. In S. Koch (Ed.), *Psychology: A study of science* (pp. 184–256). New York: McGraw Hill.

Rohnke, K. E. (1984). *Silver bullets.* Dubuque, IA: Kendall Hunt.

Rohnke, K. E. (1991). *Bottomless baggie.* Beverly, MA: Wilkscraft Creative.

Rohnke, K., E. & Butler, S. (1995). *Quicksilver.* Dubuque, IA: Kendall Hunt.

Schave, D., & Schave, B. (1989). *Early adolescence and the search for self: A developmental perspective.* New York: Praeger.

Schoel, J., & Maizell, R. (2002). *Exploring islands of healing: New perspectives on adventure based counseling.* Beverly, MA: Project Adventure.

Schoel, J., Prouty, D., & Radcliffe, P. (1988). *Islands of healing: A guide to adventure based counseling.* Beverly, MA: Project Adventure.

Thompson, C., & Henderson, D. (2006). *Counseling children* (7th ed.). Belmont, CA: Wadsworth.

Vernon, A. (2002). *What works when with children and adolescents: A handbook of individual counseling techniques.* Champaign, IL: Research Press.

Vernon, A. (2004). Working with children, adolescents, and their parents. In A. Vernon (Ed.), *Counseling children and adolescents* (3rd ed., pp. 1–34). Denver, CO: Love.

Vernon, A., & Clemente, R. (2005). *Assessment and intervention with children and adolescents: Developmental and multicultural approaches* (2nd ed.). Alexandria, VA: American Counseling Association.

Viata Training Manual. (2005). Lupeni, Romania: New Horizon.

Wampold, B. E. (2001). *The great psychotherapy debate: Models, methods, and findings.* Mahwah, NJ: Erlbaum.

Yalom, I. D. (1985). *The theory and practice of group psychotherapy* (3rd ed.). New York: Basic Books.

Yontef, G., & Jacobs, L. (2005). Gestalt therapy. In R. Corsini & D. Wedding (Eds.), *Current psychotherapies* (7th ed., pp. 299–336). Belmont, CA: Thompson/Wadsworth.

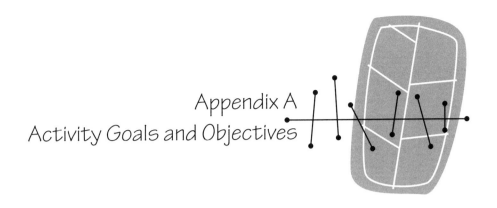

Appendix A
Activity Goals and Objectives

Goal 1: Improve Communication and Relationship Skills

Objectives:

1A. Demonstrate understanding of and apply basic communication skills (e.g., recognizing nonverbal cues, delivering "I" messages)
1B. Express feelings clearly and constructively
1C. Recognize and accept the feelings of others
1D. Express ideas clearly and constructively
1E. Listen actively to others
1F. Demonstrate willingness to trust others
1G. Develop skills for making and maintaining relationships
1H. Recognize and deal with peer pressure
1I. Use communication skills to resolve conflict
1J. Recognize the need for help and develop the ability to ask for it
1K. Recognize and verbalize needs and wishes
1L. Develop skills for effectively participating in groups

Goal 2: Increase Self-Awareness and Self-Acceptance

Objectives:

2A. Explore personal attitudes and values
2B. Identify and acknowledge personal positive traits, talents, and accomplishments
2C. Develop ability to recognize negative self-talk
2D. Develop skills in replacing negative self-talk with positive self-talk
2E. Appreciate own uniqueness
2F. Develop positive attitudes toward self
2G. Recognize personal boundaries, rights, and privacy needs
2H. Identify personal and social roles

Goal 3: Develop and Apply Problem-Solving and Decision-Making Skills

Objectives:

3A. Set personal goals
3B. Identify problems
3C. Demonstrate understanding of steps for solving problems and making decisions (gather information; explore alternatives and consequences; plan and take action)
3D. Evaluate decisions
3E. Manage change and transitions in everyday life
3F. Apply decision-making skills to resolve conflicts
3G. Apply decision-making skills in life situations
3H. Demonstrate effective coping skills for dealing with problems

3I. Recognize when peer pressure is influencing decision making

3J. Develop ability to identify alternative methods for solving problems and achieving goals

Goal 4: Increase Understanding and Valuing of Diversity

Objectives:

4A. Recognize and appreciate individual differences

4B. Develop an understanding and appreciation of own culture

4C. Demonstrate respect for others as both individuals and members of different cultural groups

4D. Acknowledge and appreciate similarities and differences across cultures and/or groups of people who have physical or learning differences

4E. Recognize how stereotypes can affect interpersonal relationships and attitudes toward others

Goal 5: Demonstrate Consistently Responsible Behavior

Objectives:

5A. Acknowledge personal responsibilities

5B. Recognize whether behavior is appropriate and responsible

5C. Act in an appropriate and responsible manner

5D. Develop coping skills for dealing with stress

5E. Understand the need for self-discipline and self-control and how to exercise them

5F. Apply time management skills

5G. Demonstrate respect for alternate perspectives

Goal 6: Enhance Positive Attitudes and Skills Related to Learning

Objectives:

6A. Develop feeling of competence and confidence as a learner

6B. Take pride in accomplishments

6C. Accept mistakes as part of the learning process

6D. Apply time management and task management strategies

6E. Recognize that effort and persistence enhance learning

6F. Demonstrate dependability and initiative

6G. Develop the ability to share knowledge

6H. Develop critical-thinking skills

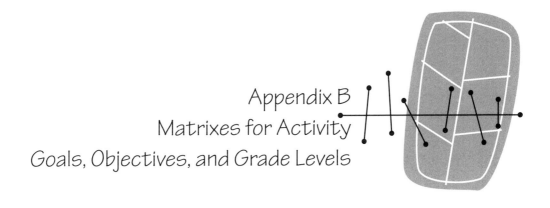

Appendix B
Matrixes for Activity
Goals, Objectives, and Grade Levels

Goal 1: Improve Communication and Relationship Skills

Activity	Minimum Grade Level	A	B	C	D	E	F	G	H	I	J	K	L
Animal Crackers	4		•	•			•	•	•	•	•		•
Bump	3		•	•	•				•	•	•		•
Carry That Load	5	•	•	•	•	•	•	•	•	•	•	•	•
Chicks and Hens	1				•		•	•			•		
Circles of Comfort	3		•	•	•	•		•	•				•
Community Puzzle	5											•	•
Cyclops Tag	3						•	•					
Electric Fence	6	•	•	•	•	•	•	•	•	•	•	•	•
Everybody Up!	2	•	•	•	•	•	•	•		•	•	•	
Guidelines	4		•	•	•	•		•	•	•			•
Hand Find	1						•	•					
Helium Stick	5	•	•	•	•	•	•	•	•	•	•	•	•
Holding It All Together	3	•			•	•		•	•	•	•	•	•
Hug Tag	1						•	•	•		•		
Human Shapes	3				•	•				•	•		•
Ice Melt	3				•				•				•
Keypunch	4		•	•	•	•			•	•	•		•
Knot or Not	1	•			•	•	•	•	•	•	•		•
Mirror Mirror	1	•						•					
Moon Ball	1	•	•	•	•	•			•	•	•	•	•
Negotiation Square	4	•	•	•	•	•			•	•	•	•	•
Paint Your Name	2								•			•	
Pass the Tire	K				•	•	•		•		•		•
Perspectives	7				•			•	•	•			•
Protect the Jewels	5				•						•	•	•
Silver Lining	3				•			•					•
Star Gate	1	•	•	•	•		•	•	•	•	•	•	•
Stretching Story	1	•	•		•	•		•			•		
Stretching the Limit	3	•			•	•			•	•		•	•
Tied Up in Knots	3	•	•	•	•	•	•	•	•	•	•	•	•
Touch My Can	3	•	•	•	•	•	•	•			•	•	•
Traffic Jam	6	•	•	•	•	•	•	•	•	•	•	•	•
Trust Walk	1	•	•	•	•	•	•	•	•		•	•	•

(Continued)

Goal 1: Improve Communication and Relationship Skills *(Continued)*

Activity	Minimum Grade Level	A	B	C	D	E	F	G	H	I	J	K	L
Turnstiles	3								•	•	•	•	•
Upchuck	5			•	•			•	•		•	•	•
Web Person	7			•	•		•	•					•
Welded Ankles	5		•	•	•	•		•	•	•	•	•	•
Yurt Pull	5		•	•		•	•	•				•	•
Zap	3		•	•									

Objectives:

A. Demonstrate understanding of and apply basic communication skills (e.g., recognizing nonverbal cues, delivering "I" messages)
B. Express feelings clearly and constructively
C. Recognize and accept the feelings of others
D. Express ideas clearly and constructively
E. Listen actively to others
F. Demonstrate willingness to trust others
G. Develop skills for making and maintaining relationships
H. Recognize and deal with peer pressure
I. Use communication skills to resolve conflict
J. Recognize the need for help and develop the ability to ask for it
K. Recognize and verbalize needs and wishes
L. Develop skills for effectively participating in groups

Goal 2: Increase Self-Awareness and Self-Acceptance

Activity	Minimum Grade Level	A	B	C	D	E	F	G	H
Animal Crackers	4	•		•	•		•		
Carry That Load	5			•	•		•	•	•
Chicks and Hens	1			•	•	•	•		•
Circles of Comfort	3	•		•	•	•			•
Community Puzzle	5		•				•	•	•
Cyclops Tag	3								•
Electric Fence	6		•	•	•	•	•	•	•
Everybody Up!	2			•	•		•	•	
Flip Me the Bird	5			•	•	•	•	•	•
Gotcha	3			•	•				
Guidelines	4	•							•
Hand Find	1			•	•	•	•		
Heads or Tails	1								•
Helium Stick	5			•	•		•	•	•
Holding It All Together	3	•							
Hug Tag	1						•		•
Human Camera	7	•	•			•	•	•	
I Can Do This!!	1		•			•			
Ice Melt	3	•	•			•	•		•
Keypunch	4		•	•	•		•		•
Known and Unknown	1	•						•	•
Mirror Mirror	1								•
Paint Your Name	2		•			•		•	
Pass the Tire	K			•	•		•	•	
Pecking Order	1	•	•	•	•		•		•
Protect the Jewels	5	•							
Silver Lining	3	•		•	•		•		
Slow Motion Tag	3			•	•	•	•	•	•
Stretching Story	1	•	•	•	•	•	•	•	•
Stretching the Limit	3						•		•
Tied Up in Knots	3		•	•	•		•		
Touch My Can	3						•		
Traffic Jam	6			•	•		•	•	
Trust Walk	1	•	•	•	•	•	•	•	•
Turnstiles	3			•	•		•		
Upchuck	5			•	•		•		•
Web Person	7		•	•	•		•	•	
Welded Ankles	5		•	•	•		•	•	•
Who Do You Follow?	5			•	•		•		•
Zap	3							•	

Objectives:

A. Explore personal attitudes and values
B. Identify and acknowledge personal positive traits, talents, and accomplishments
C. Develop ability to recognize negative self-talk
D. Develop skills in replacing negative self-talk with positive self-talk
E. Appreciate own uniqueness
F. Develop positive attitudes toward self
G. Recognize personal boundaries, rights, and privacy needs
H. Identify personal and social roles

Goal 3: Develop and Apply Problem-Solving and Decision-Making Skills

Activity	Minimum Grade Level	A	B	C	D	E	F	G	H	I	J
Animal Crackers	4					•			•	•	
Bump	3	•	•	•	•	•			•	•	•
Carry That Load	5	•	•	•	•		•	•	•	•	•
Chicks and Hens	1								•		•
Electric Fence	6	•	•	•	•	•	•	•	•	•	•
Everybody Up!	2	•	•	•							•
Heads or Tails	1				•	•		•	•	•	•
Helium Stick	5	•	•	•	•		•		•	•	•
Holding It All Together	3			•	•	•	•	•	•	•	•
Human Shapes	3		•	•	•				•	•	•
Keypunch	4	•	•	•	•		•	•	•	•	•
Knot or Not	1		•	•	•		•	•	•	•	•
Known and Unknown	1	•				•			•		•
Moon Ball	1	•	•	•	•	•	•	•	•	•	•
Negotiation Square	4	•	•	•	•		•	•	•	•	•
Pass the Tire	K								•	•	•
Protect the Jewels	5	•	•	•	•	•			•		•
Silver Lining	3					•	•		•		•
Slide Show	1					•		•	•	•	•
Star Gate	1	•	•	•	•			•	•	•	•
Star Wars Dodge Ball	1	•	•	•	•	•			•		•
Stretching the Limit	3	•							•	•	•
Tied Up in Knots	3	•	•	•	•	•	•	•	•	•	•
Touch My Can	3	•	•	•	•				•		•
Traffic Jam	6	•	•	•	•	•	•	•	•	•	•
Upchuck	5	•	•	•	•	•					•
Welded Ankles	5	•	•	•	•		•	•	•	•	•
Who Do You Follow?	5				•				•		•

Objectives:

A. Set personal goals
B. Identify problems
C. Demonstrate understanding of steps for solving problems and making decisions (gather information; explore alternatives and consequences; plan and take action)
D. Evaluate decisions
E. Manage change and transitions in everyday life
F. Apply decision-making skills to resolve conflicts
G. Apply decision-making skills in life situations
H. Demonstrate effective coping skills for dealing with problems
I. Recognize when peer pressure is influencing decision making
J. Develop ability to identify alternative methods for solving problems and achieving goals

Goal 4: Increase Understanding and Valuing of Diversity

Activity	Minimum Grade Level	A	B	C	D	E
Carry That Load	5	•	•	•	•	
Circles of Comfort	3	•	•	•	•	
Community Puzzle	5	•		•		
Electric Fence	6	•	•	•	•	•
Gotcha	3	•				
Guidelines	4	•	•	•	•	•
Hand Find	1	•	•	•	•	
Holding It All Together	3	•		•	•	
Hug Tag	1	•	•	•	•	
Human Camera	7	•	•	•	•	•
I Can Do This!!	1	•		•		•
Ice Melt	3	•	•	•	•	
Mirror Mirror	1	•	•	•	•	
Paint Your Name	2	•	•			
Pass the Tire	K	•				•
Star Gate	1	•			•	•
Stretching Story	1	•	•	•	•	•
Tied Up in Knots	3	•	•	•	•	•
Touch My Can	3	•	•		•	
Turnstiles	3	•				•

Objectives:

A. Recognize and appreciate individual differences
B. Develop an understanding and appreciation of own culture
C. Demonstrate respect for others as both individuals and members of different cultural groups
D. Acknowledge and appreciate similarities and differences across cultures and/or groups of people who have physical or learning differences
E. Recognize how stereotypes can affect interpersonal relationships and attitudes toward others

Goal 5: Demonstrate Consistently Responsible Behavior

Activity	Minimum Grade Level	A	B	C	D	E	F	G
Animal Crackers	4				•	•		
Bump	3	•			•	•		•
Carry That Load	5	•	•	•	•	•	•	•
Chicks and Hens	1			•	•	•		
Circles of Comfort	3							•
Cyclops Tag	3	•	•	•	•	•		
Electric Fence	6	•	•	•	•	•		•
Everybody Up!	2	•	•	•		•		
Flip Me the Bird	5	•	•	•	•	•		
Gotcha	3				•	•		
Hand Find	1	•	•	•	•	•		
Heads or Tails	1		•	•	•	•		
Helium Stick	5	•	•	•	•	•		•
Hug Tag	1	•	•	•	•	•		
Human Camera	7	•	•	•		•		•
Human Shapes	3				•			•
Keypunch	4	•	•	•	•	•		•
Known and Unknown	1				•	•		
Mirror Mirror	1		•	•	•	•		•
Pass the Tire	K				•	•		
Slow Motion Tag	3	•	•	•		•		
Star Gate	1				•	•		
Star Wars Dodge Ball	1	•	•	•	•	•		•
Stretching the Limit	3	•	•	•	•	•	•	•
Tied Up in Knots	3		•	•	•	•		•
Touch My Can	3	•	•	•	•	•		
Traffic Jam	6		•	•	•	•	•	
Trust Walk	1	•	•	•	•	•		
Turnstiles	3	•			•	•		
Web Person	7	•		•	•	•		
Welded Ankles	5	•	•	•	•	•		•
Yurt Pull	5	•	•	•	•	•		
Zap	3		•	•	•	•		

Objectives:

A. Acknowledge personal responsibilities
B. Recognize whether behavior is appropriate and responsible
C. Act in an appropriate and responsible manner
D. Develop coping skills for dealing with stress
E. Understand the need for self-discipline and self-control and how to exercise them
F. Apply time management skills
G. Demonstrate respect for alternate perspectives

Goal 6: Enhance Positive Attitudes and Skills Related to Learning

Activity	Minimum Grade Level	A	B	C	D	E	F	G	H
Animal Crackers	4	•	•	•		•			
Bump	3	•	•	•		•	•	•	•
Everybody Up!	2	•	•	•		•	•	•	•
Hand Find	1	•	•	•		•			•
Helium Stick	5			•				•	•
Holding It All Together	3	•				•		•	•
Human Shapes	3	•	•	•		•		•	•
Keypunch	4	•	•	•	•	•		•	•
Knot or Not	1			•				•	•
Mirror Mirror	1	•	•	•		•			
Moon Ball	1		•	•		•	•	•	•
Negotiation Square	4	•	•	•	•	•		•	•
Paint Your Name	2		•						
Pass the Tire	K		•						
Pecking Order	1	•	•	•	•	•	•		•
Perspectives	7	•	•	•	•	•	•	•	•
Slide Show	1	•	•	•	•	•	•	•	•
Star Gate	1		•	•	•	•	•	•	•
Star Wars Dodge Ball	1	•	•	•		•	•	•	•
Tied Up in Knots	3	•	•	•	•	•	•	•	•
Traffic Jam	6	•	•	•	•	•	•	•	•
Web Person	7	•	•	•	•	•	•	•	•
Welded Ankles	5		•	•	•	•	•	•	•
Who Do You Follow?	5	•	•	•					•

Objectives:

A. Develop feeling of competence and confidence as a learner
B. Take pride in accomplishments
C. Accept mistakes as part of the learning process
D. Apply time management and task management strategies
E. Recognize that effort and persistence enhance learning
F. Demonstrate dependability and initiative
G. Develop the ability to share knowledge
H. Develop critical-thinking skills

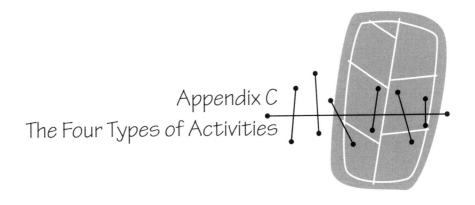

Appendix C
The Four Types of Activities

Activities by Type

Activity	Icebreaker	Deinhibitizer	Trust	Challenge/Initiative
Animal Crackers		•		
Bump		•		•
Carry That Load			•	•
Chicks and Hens		•	•	
Circles of Comfort	•	•		
Community Puzzle	•			
Cyclops Tag	•	•		
Electric Fence				•
Everybody Up!			•	•
Flip Me the Bird		•		
Gotcha	•			
Guidelines	•	•		
Hand Find	•		•	
Heads or Tails	•	•		
Helium Stick		?		•
Holding It All Together				•
Hug Tag		•		
Human Camera			•	
Human Shapes			•	•
I Can Do This!!	•	•		
Ice Melt	•			
Keypunch				•
Knot or Not		•		•
Known and Unknown	•	•		
Mirror Mirror	•			
Moon Ball		•		•
Negotiation Square		•		•
Paint Your Name	•	•		
Pass the Tire	•	•		
Pecking Order	•	•		
Perspectives				•
Protect the Jewels				•
Silver Lining	•			
Slide Show	•			
Slow Motion Tag	•			
Star Gate				•
Star Wars Dodge Ball		•		•

(Continued)

Activities by Type (Continued)

Activity	Icebreaker	Deinhibitizer	Trust	Challenge/Initiative
Stretching Story	•	•		
Stretching the Limit				•
Tied Up in Knots		•		•
Touch My Can			•	•
Traffic Jam				•
Trust Walk			•	
Turnstiles				•
Upchuck				•
Web Person			•	•
Welded Ankles				•
Who Do You Follow?		•		
Yurt Pull			•	
Zap	•			

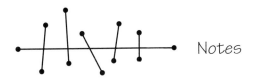 Notes

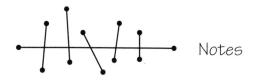 Notes

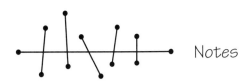

Notes

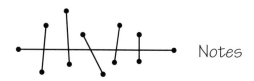

Notes